Foot Talk

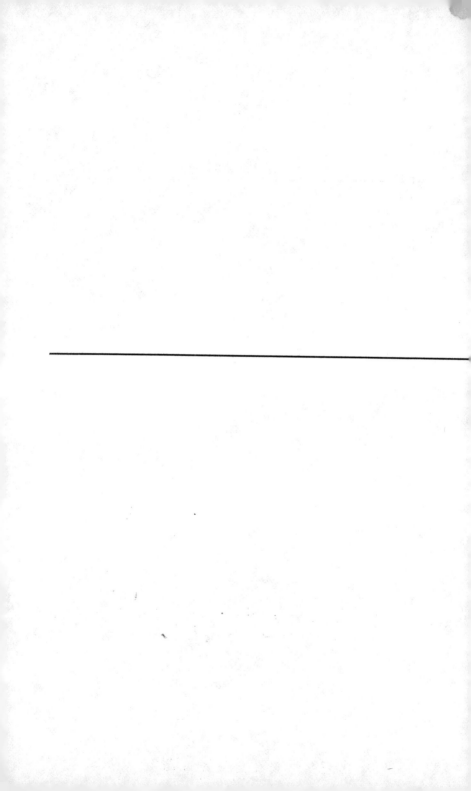

A Complete Guide to the Good Health and Care of the Feet

Foot Talk

by DR. BARRY H. BLOCK

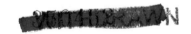
ARBOR HOUSE
NEW YORK

To my wife Hermine,
an intrinsic part of
everything I do.

Acknowledgments

I would like to thank the following foot authorities for their invaluable assistance:

Stanley Beekman, D.P.M.
Joseph D'Amico, D.P.M.
Mark Casselli, D.P.M.
Thomas DeLauro, D.P.M.
Herbert Greenberg, D.P.M.
E. Dalton McGlamry, D.P.M.
Edwin Wolf, D.P.M.

The excellent illustrations for *Foot Talk* were provided through the generosity of William Bowdler, D.P.M., Stanley Newell, D.P.M. and Peter Freund, D.P.M. and Gacci.

Special thanks to Bernard Borstein for word processing assistance.

Contents

Foot Talk

Why Talk About Feet?

1

Why talk about feet? We certainly do enough complaining about them! The feet of most active people absorb the impact of up to five million pounds every day. Try lifting just one hundred pounds with your arms and you'll understand the incredible task your feet accomplish.

But in even the most serious conversations the subject of feet invariably causes snickers. Consider a discussion recently overheard between two hospital residents:

"What field are you in?"

"I'm in podiatry."

"How can you spend all day looking at people's dirty feet?"

"Actually almost every patient's feet are clean when I examine them. What specialty are you going into?"

"Proctology."

Women in particular are very defensive about their feet. About fifty percent of my female patients enter my office saying, "Aren't these the ugliest feet you've ever seen?"

Most people think of their feet as an intimate part of their bodies. Patients are always allowed to undress their feet before the doctor enters the room. Many women who are embarrassed to take off their shoes and hosiery feel that by baring their feet they are symbolically taking off their clothes. Consider the erotic overtones of *flinging* off one's shoes.

Even general physicians shy away from examining the feet. Often a doctor will have a patient take off everything but his

1

socks and shoes. In fact, until recently most doctors received very little training in foot-related disorders.

But it cannot *all* be blamed on doctors—most of us have been guilty of neglecting our feet. *It is not normal for feet to hurt.* But we tend to tolerate pain in the feet while we won't elsewhere in the body. The too-commonly-heard phrase "my aching feet" should some day be supplemented with the expression: "When your feet hurt, you hurt all over."

Sometimes the feet do manage to get at least symbolic recognition. Outside Grauman's Chinese Theater in Hollywood, the footprints of major stars are imbedded in the concrete of the sidewalk to represent the stars themselves . . . And Cinderella would *never* have captivated the prince had her shoe size been wrong! Did you know that, like the wicked sisters of the Cinderella tale who tried to squeeze their feet into the glass slipper, over eighty percent of women today actually wear shoes that are too small for them?

The foot's role as a sex symbol reached its peak in the centuries-old Chinese practice of foot binding. Women whose feet were bound from childhood could walk only with the aid of a stick and were thus dependent on others to get around. The bound foot became a fetish for Chinese men, and young girls of five were made to suffer so that they would be revered in adulthood. The small Chinese foot was made even smaller by binding, which lifted the heel bone into an almost vertical position and permanently put the heel into a position similar to the temporary position extremely high heels create. This may sound like torture but actually it was a status symbol for a young girl to be chosen for this practice since it meant she would be spared the labors of the fields.

Various religions have long revered the foot as a symbol of humility. Consider the Pope's washing of the feet of twelve poor people on Maundy Thursday and Jesus's instruction of his disciples in the ceremony of foot washing. In Islam the feet must be washed at a fountain before entering a mosque. The Yogiis consider the foot a source of the spirit's energy.

Secular tradition has taught that it is a sign of respect—if not a mandatory practice—to kiss or bow down before the feet of monarchs.

Because shoes symbolize worldliness—and all its accompanying evils—the removal of one's shoes is an integral part of the ceremony of many religious sects. In Oriental culture one must remove his shoes before entering a house. Moses was instructed before the burning bush to "Put off thy shoes from off thy feet for the place whereon thou standest is holy ground." (Exodus 3:5)

The foot has also been the object of various forms of torture. The captured Mussolini, for example, was hung by his toes by partisan forces, and the Nazis ripped off the toenails of prisoners to secure information. A psychologically devastating practice in Islam taught that to divorce his wife, a man has merely to ceremoniously leave her shoes on his doorstep. This symbolizes his divestment of the marital relationship and its responsibilities.

All of these traditional ceremonies involving the foot and shoe have their roots in the significance of ground contact. The foot serves as our contact with the world. While we touch objects momentarily with our hands, it is our feet that have a dynamic relationship with the ground. Way back in evolutionary history the foot and hands shared a similar function and, hence, structure. In humans the hands became specialized for feeling, touching and creating, the feet for locomotion and contact with the ground.

According to Deborah Brandt, a New York body movement specialist, "Dizziness, poor self-image and even psychological disorders may have their roots in improper interaction with the ground."

Man's recognition of his relationship with the ground is demonstrated by phrases such as "Stand on your own two feet," "put your best foot forward," "get your foot in the door," and with such negative phrases as in "without a foot to stand on," "losing a foothold," and "not in step with the world."

You can tell a lot about someone by the way he walks. A nervous person tends to take short quick steps; a calmer person will take longer, slower strides. We are all familiar with the image of the anxious father-to-be, pacing the floor of a hospital waiting room. You can also tell something about a person's sexuality by the way he moves his hips or the style of shoes he wears. A swagger, high heels, pointed toes, and exposed toes are all sexual attention-getters. Does he walk with a limp? Does he move with shuffling movements like the elderly, reflecting a life of hard wear on his feet? Does he seem happy, walking with a light bouncy gait? Does he radiate confidence with his determined step? Is he stooped and walking tremulously?

Psychologists recommend walking through a dangerous area with confident strides to give the message, "I'll fight back. I'm strong." A stooped and fearful image says "I'm afraid and weak, an easy target." Consider the ominous march of soldiers in tall black boots.

Of course we are not always aware of how we walk. The physical fitness boom has at least made us more aware of our feet. But getting into shape often comes at their expense. Running and jumping, greatly magnifying the forces on our feet, has contributed directly and indirectly to countless foot injuries. Tendinitis and heel spurs are spoken of by athletes as casually as the weather. It has become almost fashionable to suffer a sport injury. But it makes a lot more sense to avoid such injuries, not only because of the pain but also because of the resulting deterioration of athletic strength.

The fitness boom has thus indirectly contributed to the increased demand for foot specialists. In 1971 only 241 students graduated from podiatry schools in the United States. By 1983 this figure had almost tripled and podiatry continues to be one of the fastest growing specialities in medicine. A 1979 Department of Health, Education and Welfare report placed podiatry as the number one health care shortage area in America. This shortage is expected to continue well into the twenty-first century.

Podiatrists go through four years of medical, surgical and orthopedic studies and often take a residency of one or more years. Athletes often use them as primary care physicians, the podiatrist referring the athlete to other specialists when necessary.

In 1964 the last degree relating to chiropody was changed to Doctor of Podiatric Medicine (D.P.M.). With this change came the training and diagnostic skills necessary to handle the medical, orthopedic and surgical needs of the foot. As foot doctors, podiatrists are trained to recognize systemic diseases and treat their manifestations in the foot. Most diabetics, for example, see a podiatrist regularly. A small abrasion on the bottom of a diabetic's foot, if left untreated, could result in a serious ulcer with devastating consequences. Before routine examination by podiatrists became customary, many diabetics had to have their feet amputated.

Podiatrists have greatly advanced the orthopedic modalities of treatment with the use of orthotics. These devices worn in the shoes compensate for structural imperfections in the foot which might otherwise have to be corrected by surgery.

The Electrodynogram®, a podiatric invention that quantifies every parameter of gait, has computerized the science of podiatric orthopedics.

In surgery, podiatrists have developed minimal-incision procedures whereby a tiny hole and a drill like a dentist's replace more traumatic large incisions made by traditional cutting instruments. This technique has earned its popularity by enabling many patients to have the surgery performed in the doctor's office, and thus avoiding expensive and time-consuming hospital stays. Laser surgery is now offered as an alternative for many procedures. Bunion reduction and the straightening out of deformed toes have been facilitated by various modern surgical procedures pioneered by podiatrists.

One of the more enduring foot fads is reflexology. With its roots in ancient Chinese and Egyptian cultures, reflexology's revival and popularity can be attributed to Eunice Stopfel, whose 1968 book *Reflexology Chart—Relation of the Body to the Feet* gained popularity with the health and nutrition boom.

Remember the adage "If your foot hurts, you hurt all over"? If you extend the thought, pain in another part of the body becomes linked with an inadequacy of the foot. Reflexologists claim that crystal like deposits in the feet cause congestion and dysfunction in specific organs. By massaging different areas of the foot, reflexologists say they are able to free the transmission of energy to the specific organ involved, reestablishing normal function therein. These claims have not been proved nor have they held up to medical testing, but the massage probably does make you feel better.

The feet are not islands of abuse. They are the foundation upon which our bodies operate. Think of it in terms of the old song: "The foot bone's connected to the leg bone and the leg bone's connected to the thigh bone" and so on—all the way up

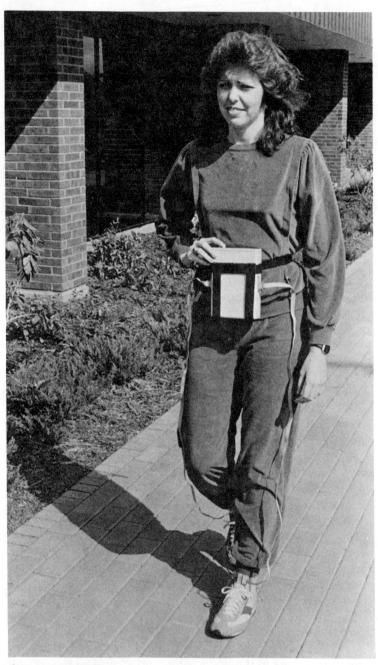

Gait analysis done using an Electrodynagram® (courtesy of Langer Biomechanics Group, Deer Park, N.Y.)

to the torso. When you suffer from a foot problem, the resultant trauma will travel up the leg to the knee, hip and back. I can't tell you how often people call my office with foot complaints, mentioning as an aside that they are experiencing pain in their knees. And yet they don't seem to make the connection between one pain and the other.

Less obvious is the connection between foot and back pain. "Gee doc, these backaches I've been having for years can't be related to my feet. My feet just started hurting me." Upon questioning the patient, this last statement proves not to be the case. "Of course my feet hurt at the end of the day. That's normal, isn't it?"

No. You may be able to ignore the pain but your body structure will not be able to ignore the trauma causing the pain. It is unlikely that you will have a foot problem without having other related structural problems.

The foot is a compensatory organ, forced to adapt to any structural imperfections in the skeleton. If your body's equilibrium is ever disturbed by a limp, for even a short period of time, you'll notice the effects on your entire body. Your legs, hips, back, shoulders and arms will be thrown off balance as the feet compensate for the injured part. Muscles unaccustomed to bearing the added strain will start to ache.

Many people think that foot problems are inherited. Your mother had a bunion as did her mother, and therefore you are convinced that no matter what, your developing bunion cannot be prevented. While it is true that genetics does play a vital role in what we have to work with, there is also a great deal that one can do today to compensate for structural problems. In the case of a bunion, for instance, the wearing of an orthotic device counteracts the forces that caused the formation of your mother's bunion. If you have a strong family history of a particular foot problem, and you find that you are developing symptoms of that problem, you should see a foot specialist immediately. Often conditions such as hammertoes and heel spurs can be prevented before surgery becomes necessary—but time is *not* on your side. It is a good idea to bring your children with you to have the doctor examine them. He may be able to see an underlying pathology before any symptoms become evident. Unfortunately, most structural foot problems develop so slowly that they are not detected. By the time there is foot pain, surgery may be necessary.

Shoes play only a partial but significant role in creating deformed and painful feet. Too often the shoe conforms not to the outline of the foot but to a designer's stylized conception of how the foot should look. This takes on its actual form in the wooden last (a mold used by shoemakers, around which shoes are built). The last is generally symmetrical as is the resulting shoe *but*— (have designers not noticed?)—the foot is not symmetrical! From the shoe buying habits of women it would seem that they would sooner alter their feet to fit the shoe than wear the shoe that fits.

To walk comfortably in today's fantasies of fashion, one's middle toe would have to be the "big toe" flanked by two smaller toes on each side.

When Japanese women started wearing western-style shoes, they actually had to learn to walk in them and often resorted to illustrations akin to the diagrams we use for learning a new dance.

Consider the irony of mothers running out to buy their infants shoes to speed up or enhance their walking. Aside from the fact that these early shoes cause discomfort, they also do not permit babies to stretch their toes, to experience their environment. Almost always the walking of these early shod babies is impeded, and occasionally serious damage is done to the foot structure.

It is not only our shoes that test the foot's endurance—socks play their part in this effort as well. The ideal stocking would be a lightweight, breathable absorbent cotton covering with digital appendages exactly fitting each toe. Such footwear was actually once sold throughout the United States. If you have difficulty finding a shoe that fits, think how complicated it would be to find your digital sock size! In the next chapter we will examine footwear buying habits and show you how to best find the shoe that fits.

Shoes: You Are What You Wear

2

If your shoes could talk, they would sound a lot like you! Their style, color, heel height, and ornamentation all reflect your personality and lifestyle. Think about the kind of shoes *you* buy. What colors do you choose and what heel height do you select? What are they saying to the outside world? Do you buy shoes for fashion or comfort?

Compare the sexy, red, high-heeled, pointed-toe slingback shoe worn by an attractive 25-year-old single woman to the dull brown "sensible" orthopedic type oxford worn by an elderly widow. What messages are they conveying? The young woman is interested in attracting the eye of men. Her shoes are saying "look at me." The older woman is not looking for attention. Her shoes are saying "leave me alone, I want to be comfortable." Many women whose feet scream out for comfortable shoes actually won't buy them because they fear the symbolic loss of youth, style, and fashion.

The expensive designer shoe of the executive woman on her way up whispers success . . . and the motorcycle gang member's heavy black boot shows hostility.

Your shoes also reflect the state of the economy and the current socio-political climate. Remember the shoes of the turbulent sixties and early seventies? Shoe styles were unconventional. Sleek classic lines were replaced by thick and chunky platform shoes. Flower children wore tie-dyed tennis sneakers. Unisex styles underscored the women's liberation movement's demand for sexual equality. Compare those shoes to the preceding boom years of the late fifties when pointed-toe stiletto high heels were the rage, or to the low-heeled pumps in the early eighties, reflecting a recessionary economy and a return to conservative values. What will future shoe styles be like? Many shoe designers profess to set the fashion trends. In reality, most of them merely follow the latest fad.

Thousands of new shoe styles are introduced each year. The ones that succeed often do so because the economic and social conditions are ripe for their acceptance. In recessionary times, people buy fewer shoes. Practicality becomes more of an influence. In boom years, people buy more shoes and we see the emergence of more radical styles.

Though not following the natural contours of the foot, the pointed-toe shoe has through the years proven itself the most sexually explicit and popular of all shoe styles. It gives the foot a trim, alluring look and slenderizes an anatomically stubby forefoot. In 1948 designers reintroduced pointed-toe shoes, but they were a dismal flop. The post-war recession made the public conservative and they were simply not ready for them. Why were these same pointed-toe shoes so popular from the mid-fifties to the early sixties? The economy was booming and people were abandoning their conservative values and dress styles.

Sometimes a style is tied to a revered public figure. Count Alfred Guillaume Gabriel d'Orsay (1801–1852), one of the most flamboyant socialites of mid-nineteenth century Europe, designed a pump shoe with cutout sides which rapidly became the rage of the continent. The "sensible" orthopedic-looking oxford shoes of the twenties and thirties were greatly popularized by our first lady, Eleanor Roosevelt, who firmly believed that foot comfort was more important than style.

Fashion

But fashion, not comfort, has consistently been the primary factor in determining shoe styles. And because fashion is always changing, you can be sure that whatever trend is now popular won't be for long. William A. Rossi is a former podiatrist and currently serves as a consultant to the footwear industry. In his book *The Sex Life of the Foot and Shoe* he related the story of a woman telling her psychiatrist of a disturbing dream—she was walking down the street naked, except for her shoes. "And you felt deeply embarrassed?" probed her psychiatrist. "Terribly so," she replied, "they were last year's shoes."

A popular misconception is that the primary function of shoes is to support and protect the feet. Historically, Rossi places these utilitarian uses behind those of fashion and status.

Originally all shoes were designed for men. It is only in recent times that female styles have become the trend setters.

Each year over thirty thousand new styles reach American shoe stores and women's shoe styles account for over seventy-five percent of them. Is it only coincidence that over seventy-five percent of all podiatry patients are female?

Each of these styles stems from only seven basic shoe types:

MOCCASIN (12,000 B.C.)—The oldest of all shoes, originally a piece of hide wrapped around the foot.

SANDAL (7,000 B.C.)—This basic shoe is still popular, especially in Mediterranean countries. The word sandal is derived from the Latin "sanis," meaning a thong attached to a board of leather.

MULE (2,500 B.C.)—A backless slipper, the word mule is derived from the Sumerian word "mulu" meaning indoor shoe.

BOOT (1000 A.D.)—This started out as a separate legging attachment to a shoe. Eventually the boot evolved into a shoe type all its own, providing a popular location for pirates to stash their contraband. This practice gave rise to the expression "bootlegged."

MONK (1400 A.D.)—A low cut slip-on shoe with a wide strap crossing the instep, this shoe was designed by an Alpine monk and was popular in European monasteries. The universally popular clog, a wooden-soled shoe, is a derivative of the monk. In Japan they are known as getas and in Europe as sabots. During the industrial revolution, disgruntled European workers threw their shoes into the new machinery giving rise to the word "sabotage."

PUMP (1540 A.D.)—Today's most popular female shoe, it was originally a low cut slipper to which a heel was added. The name is derived from the "pumps," or car-

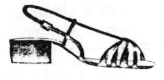

Sandal

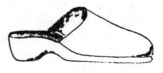

Mule

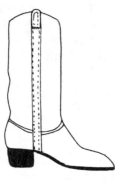

Boot

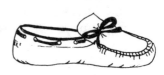

Moccasin

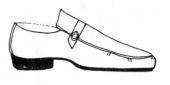

Monk Strap

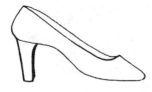

Pump

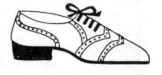

Oxford

From All About Shoes *(The Footwear Council)*

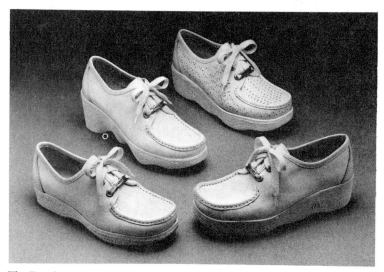

The Famolare wave sole shoe

riage drivers of nineteenth century Europe, who found this shoe comfortable for pumping the hydraulic mechanism used in the operation of the carriage.

OXFORD (1640 A.D.)—This sturdy laced-up shoe gets its name from its place of origin: Oxford, England. This shoe, popular among Oxford's collegians, was inspired by the laced corset and surprisingly didn't make its debut in America until the turn of the twentieth century.

Modern styles are either combinations or direct offshoots of the above. A loafer, for example, is an offshoot of the mocassin. Joe Famolare, designer of the unique four wave sole shoe, often combines elements of a monk (clog) with either a sandal, pump, or oxford.

Status

Shoes have always reflected status. In ancient Roman and Greek civilizations, shoe types could often be used to differentiate class. Only the nobility and soldiers wore sandals. The poorer

Poulaines (From All About Shoes, *The Footwear Council)*

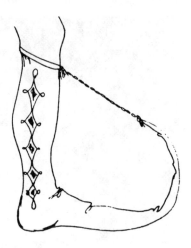

classes and slaves went barefoot in the streets. Courtesans often wore soles studded with nails arranged to spell "follow me."

In Greek drama, actors wore platform shoes called korthonos. The more important the actor and his role, the higher the platform on his shoe. In ancient Oriental culture, not even the nobility wore shoes. Only the Emperor wore shoes and even he removed them when praying to the gods. It was considered an insult to wear shoes before the Emperor, and thus began the custom of removing your shoes before entering an Oriental house.

Poulaines were extended-point shoes popular in thirteenth to fifteenth century Europe. Government regulations established the maximum permissible length of the tip according to class. Commoners were restricted to six inches, gentlemen a foot, and noblemen two feet or more. Kings and princes of course, could wear any length they desired.

By the sixteenth century, shoe styles had changed so that width replaced length as a status symbol. The Italian scarpine was known in England as the duckbill. Queen Mary, during her reign (1553–1558) found it necessary to limit the maximum width to six inches.

Even today, shoes are a sign of success. From a park bench in Manhattan's Central Park you can tell a lot about people by their shoes. Secretaries and tellers usually don't wear three-hundred-dollar Maud Frizon shoes, but their female bosses often do.

There's the well worn basic work shoe of the blue collar worker versus the highly polished wingtip Bally worn by the top executive. Shoes may not make the man, but they have a lot to say about his success.

Heel Heights

One of the most controversial features of any shoe is the heel height. This too follows a cyclical pattern. High heels and platforms go back thousands of years. Archaeologists opened a tomb in Thebes and discovered platform shoes with twelve-inch heels. Heel height actually peaked in fifteenth century Europe. Aristocratic Italian women wore heels with an average length of six to eighteen inches. These shoes, known as chopines, were sometimes as high as stilts (thirty inches) and were considered so dangerous that a Venice law of 1430 prohibited their use by pregnant women. Fashion, though, was considered so important that women still risked the life of an unborn child to stay in style.

For short men, heel height is of special significance. Sociologists today confirm the importance of overall height. Elevator shoes with a hidden heel have long been popular with shorter men. Sylvester Stallone of "Rocky" fame wears them. Can you imagine a heavyweight champion being only 5 feet 7 inches tall?

For women, heel height is much more a measure of sensuality and sexiness. The high heel tends to modify the posture for that long, leggy look and transform an awkward looking perpendicular foot into a pointed extension of the leg. It also creates the illusion that the foot is smaller and has a higher arch. Functionally, high heels shorten gait and accentuate hip movement. Rossi calls this the "bondage gait" and points out that many men find this unsure "dependent" gait of the high-heeled woman attractive because it makes *them* feel more masculine. Rossi concludes that the "willow walk" created by the binding of Chinese women's feet represents another form of male domination. Sexual researchers from Freud to Ellis and Kinsey have all recognized the sexual allure of high heels.

On the other end of the spectrum are negative heel shoes. Anna Kelso's Earth Shoe® of the late sixties was a dramatic and unsuccessful version of this concept that eventually turned out to be the "Edsel" of the industry. Part of the Earth Shoe's perceived ugliness came from its natural foot-shaped appearance which rendered the forepart of the shoe extremely comfortable. The real weakness of the shoe was its lack of heel height. Kelso failed to appreciate the evolutionary importance of an adequate heel. Humans have simply not yet adapted from our tree dwelling ape-like past to today's ground surfaces. The evolutionary pattern of other mammals that have made the transition to ground surfaces has been to rise up on their forefoot (much like a cat or a horse). This increases the mechanical advantage of the foot and thus increases running speed. To walk properly, the leg must move over the ankle, causing the foot to dorsi-flex (picture your toes coming toward your nose). Most humans have a shortening of their calf muscles, which limits this motion. By adding a small heel lift, the effective range of motion of the ankle becomes increased, and walking becomes easier.

The low heels of the early eighties were a result of the fitness boom, with an increase in designer sneaker and dance-inspired shoes. Recessionary times and a return to conservative values has also had an effect on the shoe industry.

High heels—though always the target of consumer-oriented health groups, including podiatrists—are destined to return. We hear over and over that they cause foot problems by increasing pressure on the forefoot and that they increase the chances of falling. There's no disputing the validity of these statements. But do they have any effect on the shoe buying habits of women or the design concepts of the shoe industry? Of course not! Women will continue to be interested in wearing fashionable shoes and the shoe industry interested in selling to them.

In search of a fashionable yet comfortable shoe, I visited New York City's elegant Maud Frizon showroom. Most of the styles were gorgeous, but not, in my opinion, suitable for human feet. Finally, I discovered a low-heeled stylish pump with an adequate toe box. I congratulated the salesman on the beautiful yet comfortable shoe. "Sir," he sniffed, "Maud Frizon shoes are designed for fashion; comfort is secondary."

Women are almost always willing to suffer foot pain in the name of fashion. A young actress once complained to me that her feet were killing her. My examination revealed no structural problems—her stylish shoes simply did not match her feet. When I suggested that she try a semi-fashionable Revelation, she looked horrified. "I wouldn't be caught dead in those." And she meant it!

Psychologists dub this phenomena algolagnia, pain with pleasure or pleasure from pain. This form of podo-masochism is routinely endured by millions of women daily. It is a price willingly paid.

Men are less likely to pay this price. There is, however the classic story of a distressed man who complained to his shoe salesman, "My life is miserable. I'm hen-pecked by my wife. My daughter ran away with a gigolo, and my son gives me grief. If only I could have one moment of pleasure." The salesman proceeded to bring the man a pair of size-seven shoes. "But you know I wear size nine," the man exclaimed. "I know," quipped the salesman, "but after a whole day of wearing these, imagine the pleasure you'll feel when you take them off!"

The whole concept of properly fitting shoes needs to be debunked. Except for custom molded shoes, no shoe can ever be expected to fit everyone properly. How can they? No two pair of feet are identical. In fact, each foot is slightly different. Shoes are constructed over a model called a last, which resembles a foot. Actually, a last represents the shoe designer's illusion of what a foot *should* look like. Take a close look at your foot and you'll notice it tends to be particularly wide in the front part near the bases of the big and little toes. This is aesthetically unappealing. The shoe designer's last tries to eliminate this unsightly line and provide a graceful curve to the front of the shoe. Without this curve you would wind up with a sexless, "sensible" shoe which would be functionally comfortable.

Lasts were originally chiseled out of stone. For thousands of years they were carved out of wood. Only since 1961 have they been made out of plastic. The transition to plastic was important because it created a uniformity in lasts by eliminating the warping which occurred in wood.

Another problem in finding a proper fitting shoe is that each manufacturer uses his own lasts and may even change them from time to time. There is no guarantee that if your foot measures a size 7B that any 7B will fit perfectly, not even a 7B from your favorite manufacturer.

Sizes

American and English shoe sizes originated in 1324, when the English King Edward II declared that three barleycorns equaled one inch. He determined that the largest possible foot was thirteen inches (thirty-nine barleycorns). Thus was the origin of men's size thirteen. By this formula, we can calculate size by measuring foot length. Each size up or down from thirteen is an additional one-third inch, each half-size one-sixth inch.

If your foot is twelve inches long, theoretically you should wear a size ten, if your foot is eleven and five-sixths inches, you would wear size nine-and-a-half. Of course, it is necessary to know your size, but you should judge a shoe on the basis of comfort. A well-fitting new shoe should feel like an "old" shoe.

Most countries of the world are on the metric system, where sizes are based on centimeters (1 inch = 2.54 cm).

What's Your Shoe Buying I.Q.?

We generally have an idea of the type of shoe we set out to buy. A walking shoe, an elegant evening slingback, a sports shoe. We often plan on color, style, and even on a particular department store to purchase our shoes. Our shoe buying habits, however, often do not include other important considerations. Take this test to evaluate your shoe buying I.Q.

---

1. When is the proper time to buy shoes?
   a) first thing in the morning
   b) at the end of the day
   c) on your day off

2. In choosing your shoes, what materials do you look for?
   a) natural materials
   b) synthetic materials such as naugahyde and vinyl
   c) it makes no difference

3. For most people the heel height of a good walking shoe is:
   a) three inches
   b) a flat shoe
   c) one to two inches

Size chart comparing American to French and metric shoe sizes (Sterling Last Company)

4. If a shoe store does not have the style you want in your proper width you:
   a) should find a store that does
   b) can take a narrower width providing you buy shoes a half-size longer
   c) have the salesman stretch out the shoe

5. In "breaking in" a shoe you should:
   a) wear it as long as possible
   b) wear it for short intervals for several days
   c) keep them in shoe trees for a few days before wearing them

6. When you buy shoes it is best to:
   a) wear them home to break them in
   b) take them home and wear them around the house first
   c) waterproof them before you wear them

7. A shoe should be flexible
   a) in the back
   b) in the front
   c) all over

8. For support, shoes should be rigid:
   a) at the toe area
   b) at the counter or back of the shoe
   c) all over

9. For good arch support "cookies," prefabricated foam inserts, are:
   a) very effective
   b) completely ineffective
   c) somewhat effective

10. Sending for shoes from a mail-order catalog:
    a) is recommended only if you are sure of your size
    b) is wise only if you are instructed to send a tracing of your foot
    c) is never recommended

Answer Key—Shoe Buying IQ			
1.	B	6.	B
2.	A	7.	B
3.	C	8.	B
4.	A	9.	C
5.	B	10.	C

Buying Shoes

Buying shoes requires common sense. I do not recommend that you buy from a catalog because, as previously mentioned, each manufacturer has his own concept of what a particular size should be, and even this can change. Some mail-order houses try to get around this problem by asking you to send them a tracing of your foot along with your order. Unfortunately, this is only of limited value. Even if correct, a tracing provides only a two-dimensional representation of a three-dimensional foot. There is simply no better way to buy a shoe than at a large well-stocked shoe store. There you'll have the opportunity to try on many different sizes.

In many individuals, one foot is slightly larger than the other. In this case, always buy the shoe for the largest foot and have the salesman fill in the shoe of the smaller foot with felt or moleskin.

Your shoe size will not stay constant throughout your life. While your foot completes most of its growth by the age eighteen or twenty its size might increase if the arch collapses, which results in a wider, longer foot.

The best time to shop for shoes is after work when the feet are generally swollen to their maximum. Have you ever bought a shoe which felt great in the store, only to find out the next day that it was tight? Chances are you bought the shoe too early in the day. Remember, your feet are the lowest part of the body and as the day progresses, gravity causes fluids to accumulate there.

Materials

Leather is the best material to look for in a shoe. It is also one of the most expensive because it is derived from animal skins. These skins then undergo a process known as tanning and emerge as leather. Suede and patent leather receive additional processing to achieve their characteristic look and feel.

In addition to its rich look and feel, leather has many advantages over less expensive synthetic vinyls. It is more breathable, which allows perspiration (ninety-eight percent water and two percent salt) to escape from your shoes. The salt acts as a corrosive agent which causes the decomposition of the shoe. External salt, used to melt ice in winter, is also an enemy of your

22   **Foot Talk**

shoes. Wash off this salt as soon as possible with a solution of
one pint of water and one teaspoon of vinegar.

Leather shoes will last longer and look better if they are properly cared for. This requires periodic cleaning, waxing and po-
lishing. The use of wooden shoe trees is recommended to maintain the shape of your shoes. Stuffing your shoes with crumpled
newspaper is another good idea, particularly after a shoe has
been exposed to wetness.

Finding the Proper Size

Never accept a different size or width than the one you need. A
7B is not the same as a 7½A. If they were, why would the
manufacturer produce both sizes? Shoe salesmen are out to
make a living, and many just don't care if you have a few extra
problems adapting to a new shoe.

For proper sizing, first compare your sole to the bottom of the
shoe. The widest part of your foot (near the ball) should correspond to the widest part of the shoe.

Now stand up with the shoe on. You should be able to easily
wiggle your toes. If you can't, either the shoe is too short or the
toe box is too low. If your toes are hammered or you have a
tendency to develop corns, you'll need a shoe with a high toe
box.

Do not accept the salesman's statement that a snug shoe will
stretch. There is no guarantee of this. A properly fitting shoe
should feel comfortable the first time you try it on. Even if a shoe
does stretch, it may be at the expense of your feet. "If the shoe
fits, wear it" is all well and good, but remember, too, if the shoe
doesn't fit, don't buy it.

Never wear new shoes home. If they don't fit properly,
chances are they will be too worn to return them to the store.
Breaking in a new shoe should be done at short intervals inside.
During this process, the foot actually molds the shoe. Did you
know that before the nineteenth century there were virtually no
right or left shoes? One bought two identical shoes. The shoe
you wore on the right foot became molded and became the right
shoe. The left was molded in a similar manner. This process was
often painful, yet accepted. In 1839, a Philadelphia craftsman

introduced right and left shoes and was dubbed the "crooked shoemaker." After a while his idea gained popularity and by the twentieth century all shoes were made in rights and lefts. Because your foot molds a shoe to its own shape, you should not wear someone else's shoe, even if it is the correct size.

Proper Heel Height

The proper heel height is the *lowest* one that you can wear comfortably. Your foot structure and the length of your calf muscle will dictate which height is best for you. If you can't touch your toes from a standing position with your knees straight, your calf muscles are short and you'll need a higher heel. If you can touch your toes easily, you'll probably be more comfortable in a flatter shoe.

A good walking shoe generally has a heel ranging from one to two inches. Dressier shoes generally range from two inches up. The wider the heel, the more stability you're going to get. A flat shoe, while being quite stable, can often cause knee pain. Athletic shoe manufacturers have gradually increased the height of the heels on sport shoes to prevent this problem. The flat sneaker (pre-1970) became obsolete during the fitness boom of the seventies and eighties. Its lack of heel resulted in too many cases of knee pain and Achilles tendinitis.

Support

Look for support in whatever shoe you buy. Shoes often receive extra support by the addition of a steel shank. Usually found in more expensive shoes, this shank is a flat piece of metal running from the heel to the arch area and its specific function is to support the arch and to prevent the shoe from collapsing under your body's weight. Some shoes such as the espadrille and the clog do not require a shank because the area under the arch is already filled in.

Arch supports or "cookies" are small prefabricated pads built into the arch area of a shoe. They are often made of foam rubber and are limited in their ability to provide support. If you need arch support, you'll be far better off visiting your podiatrist who can customize specific devices for your particular foot.

The counter or back of the shoe should be "stiff" to provide additional stability and support for the shoe. If you can easily bend this part, look for another shoe. Backless shoes are non-supportive and not recommended for heavy individuals. Continual wearing of backless shoes often results in the formation of heel fissures (painful cracks in the skin around the heel).

Flexibility

The only part of the shoe which should be flexible is the forepart, which must flex to permit normal walking. Always test to make sure you can easily flex the shoe near the area of the ball of the foot.

Shock Absorption

The pavement and floors of today's cities are hard on your feet. Forces not adequately absorbed by your shoes pass uninterrupted to your knees, hips, and lower back. It's no small wonder that people who move from a rural to an urban area often find themselves visiting the podiatrist far more often. Most shoe manufacturers are unfortunately too cost-conscious to provide the adequate inner cushioning we desperately need. If your feet are often sore at the end of the day, you should buy a pair of either Spenco insoles (nitrogen-inpregnated foam) or PPT insoles (porometric foam). Although these insoles are more expensive than the foam type sold in drugstores, they are a better value. They are washable and far more shock-absorbent than the disposable type foam insoles.

A rubber or crepe sole provides the best external shock absorption. If they are thick enough, leather soles can provide an adequate degree of shock absorption. This is seldom the case with high style shoes. Wood is occasionally used as a sole and as you might expect, is unacceptable as a shock absorber. Generally, polyurethane soles provide the best combination of shock absorption and wear and are the most widely used today.

Boots

The three basic types of boots are fashion boots (generally made of thin leather), casual boots (of a more durable leather), and foul weather boots (water-proofed or water-resistant).

Foul weather boots, particularly popular in medieval Europe when the streets were unpaved, muddy, and often strewn with garbage, provide the best protection from the elements.

Boots should be removed when you arrive at your home or office. While they keep moisture from getting in, they also prevent it from leaving, causing your feet to become particularly sweaty.

Boots and shoes should not be worn on consecutive days. The accumulated moisture should be given adequate time to evaporate and dry thoroughly. Excessive moisture in your shoes creates an unhealthy environment for your feet. Bacteria, fungi, yeast, and mold all thrive in the warm, dark, moist climate of a shoe. This moisture may take several days to completely evaporate. Ideally, you should have a different pair of shoes for every day of the week.

If you must wear shoes on consecutive days, use a hair dryer, set on medium, for a few minutes to dry out the shoe. It's best to avoid the high setting since too rapid a drying will shrink the leather of the shoe. Leaving a shoe near a heater is likewise not recommended. If you don't have a hair dryer, you can stuff your shoes with newspaper.

Adding cornstarch to your shoes is another effective way to keep them dry. Cornstarch is preferable to talc because it absorbs many times the moisture and talc has been found to contain some dangerous impurities such as asbestos. The only caution with using powders is that they can sometimes be messy.

Orthopedic and Corrective Shoes

One of the most controversial of all shoe topics is whether orthopedic shoes are of any value. Generally these shoes are solidly built oxfords with one or more of the following features.

1. THOMAS HEEL   This is a heel which is extended forward to the instep and intended to provide additional support against

excessive pronation (the collapsing of the arch). The problem with the Thomas Heel is that any support it once provided has been lost as the size of the heel extension has decreased over the years.

2. ROCKER BAR OR FORWARD THRUST   This is an extra lump added to the sole of the shoe at the ball area (where the shoe usually flexes). This causes the foot to "rock" forward, thus eliminating motion at the metatarsophalangeal joints. A rocker bar added to a shoe can be useful in decreasing pain in individuals suffering from severe arthritis of the feet. Be especially careful when climbing stairs while in a forward thrust or rocker shoe— it's possible for the sole extension to get caught on a rung of the stair and trip you.

3. CUBOID, NAVICULAR, AND METATARSAL PADS   These are pre-fabricated inserts designed to fit under a specific part of the foot. Unfortunately, they probably won't exactly match your foot and as a result may actually cause more pain than they relieve.

Not enough solid research is available to resolve the controversy over the value of orthopedic shoes. Such research, however, does support the wearing of orthotic devices (see Chapter Six). Orthotics are custom-made inserts which are designed to fit in shoes. Because they are made from a specific casting of your foot, they will match your foot exactly, and provide support where you need it. Orthotics can be worn in most closed shoes and sneakers and thus look better and are a far better value than orthopedic shoes. Studies have shown that orthotics can modify gait and decrease orthopedically based pain.

Molded Shoes

Molded or "space shoes" are custom-made shoes which are indicated for those with severely deformed or unusually sized or shaped feet (when your feet are of different sizes, for example, and mass produced shoes cannot be comfortably worn). To make them, a shoemaker uses plaster to make a last of your foot over which the shoe can be built. Although expensive, these shoes are generally extremely comfortable.

Do Shoes Cause Structural Foot Problems?

This is a controversial subject. Citing anthropologists' observations of bunions among the unshod peoples of the world, some experts contend that shoes have little or no effect on the formation of foot problems of this nature. Others argue that shoes are responsible for *all* structural foot problems.

The truth lies somewhere between the two extremes. The tendency to form most structural conditions is hereditary. If your foot is intrinsically unstable and nothing is done to correct the condition, you will probably develop foot problems, regardless of what shoe you wear. The wearing of improperly shaped or sized shoes will accelerate this process. Pointed shoes, for instance, act as a deforming force on the forefoot. The more stable your joints are, the less likely they will be deformed by wearing pointed toe shoes. Two people with different foot types will react differently to the same shoe: the unstable foot may form a bunion rapidly and the stable foot may resist the deforming force of the shoes for years.

Socks and Hosiery

Your choice of hosiery can markedly influence your foot health. The nylon hose most commonly worn by women may be attractive, but it is not a very breathable material. Over a half pint of fluid secreted by each foot every day must be allowed to evaporate through your shoes and socks. If your feet tend to sweat, it's a good idea to wear cotton hose or socks whenever possible. If you must wear nylons, get into the habit of carrying an extra pair, so that you can change them during the day.

Today, nylon hosiery is manufactured with built-in obsolesence. As any woman knows, the slightest encounter with a sharp toenail or desk edge invariably leads to a tear.

Manufacturers have long possessed the technology to produce virtually indestructable hose. During World War II, nylons were produced which lasted for months or longer. Too long, in fact, for the hosiery industry to make the kind of "turnover" profit they knew a more "fragile" hose would produce. It's unlikely that truly runless hosiery will be sold unless the public demands it.

In general natural materials such as cotton and wool are far better for your feet because natural fibers provide a "wicking" effect which absorbs moisture and keeps the feet cool as your perspiration rapidly evaporates.

Climate should also be a factor in selecting socks. In warm weather, an all-cotton or high cotton content sock is best. In cold weather, wool socks provide the best combination of insulation and "wicking" If you don't tolerate wool well, an acceptable alternative is an eighty-five percent orlon, fifteen percent cotton blend.

A final note about socks. A popular misconception is that white socks are superior to colored socks because they contain no dye. Inevitably when a patient comes into my office with an infection he is wearing white socks because he assumes that they are "sterile." But what most people don't know is that today even white socks contain dye. And in fact there is no evidence that white socks are better for your feet than colored socks.

Your shoes and hosiery reflect your lifestyle and fashion. Whether you wear an exotic high-heel shoe with black nylon hose or a sensible oxford with white cotton socks, you're providing a home for your feet—try to make it as comfortable and healthy as possible.

By The Skin Of Your Feet

3

Let your imagination run wild: you're stuffed into a suitcase that's being tossed around all day. You're hot and sweaty, barely able to breathe. There's no relief in sight.

Not a comfortable picture . . . but a pretty fair representation of what the skin of your feet has to cope with every day. No wonder the first thing many people do when they arrive home is to take off their shoes. Ah, the fresh air. The pleasure.

Considering the fact that your feet must live in an environment that would violate the Geneva Convention, it's not surprising that skin problems constitute the number one reason patients see a podiatrist. Most of these problems are either preventable or curable.

The skin of the sole is a marvel of dermatology, different from skin everywhere else on the body (except the palms). It is ten times the thickness of normal skin. Despite the protection afforded by this layer, many friction-related disorders often result.

Corns and Calluses

Among the most common afflictions of the feet are corns and calluses. And they have been around for thousands of years. In Shakespeare's *Romeo and Juliet*, Capulet declares "Welcome gentlemen! ladies that have their toes unplagu'd with corns . . . which of you all will now deny to dance? She that makes dainty, she, I'll swear hath corns."

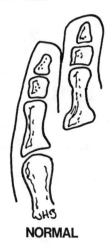
NORMAL

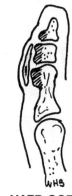
HARD CORN
with bone deformity

The English words "corn" and "callus" are derived from the Latin *cornu* meaning horn and *callus* meaning hard skin. Corns and calluses are accumulations of dead skin which are created by the body to protect the underlying foot bones and structures from excessive trauma. Abnormal stresses such as friction stimulate the skin to grow faster than the body can shed it off. Corns and calluses have no "roots," nor are they contagious.

Callus forms over diffuse areas such as the ball of the foot or the heel. Corns develop over smaller precise locations such as on or between toes. It is possible to form corns on the bottom of the foot or even under a toenail, but it is unlikely that a callus will form on or between toes.

The friction that stimulates most corn and callus formation generally occurs when the skin finds itself squeezed between the shoe on the outside and a foot bone on the inside. Often an underlying bursa is associated with a corn. These balloon-like sacs fill up with fluid to further cushion the underlying bones. There is certainly a sound basis for the old wives' tale that people with corns can predict an upcoming storm. When the barometer drops, the atmospheric pressure decreases, which causes the fluid in the bursa below a corn to expand, thus making the corn even more painful. If your corns hurt more during bad weather or if you experience pain when the sides of your corn are squeezed, you probably have an inflammed bursa underneath your corn.

Initially, the corn or callus serves a useful function in that it toughens the skin. If, however, the cause of the problem (either the ill-fitting shoe and/or the underlying bone) is not corrected, the lesion will grow and after a while, the corn or callus will be so large that instead of protecting the foot, it will cause pain. Many times corns have a central core or eye, which is known as the radix. This area lies directly over the offending bony prominence or spur.

Try an experiment. Take a tiny pebble and place it into the bottom of your shoe. Now try walking. That's how painful a corn can be. Calluses create a different type of pain, usually described as burning or aching.

Prevention

The easiest way to prevent corns is to wear only properly fitting shoes. If your feet don't rub against the inside of the shoe, it's doubtful you'll ever develop a corn. If your shoes are too narrow, you may even develop corns between your toes. These annoying and painful lesions are known as "soft" corns, aptly named, because they are located in the moistened interspace of your toes, where they become macerated and soft.

Wearing a wide shoe prevents external pressure from causing a corn to form. Elective toe surgery prevents the corn internally. If your lifestyle or occupation requires you to wear stylish or pointed-toe shoes, an in-office procedure (see Chapter Eleven) can easily eliminate the underlying bony prominence causing the corn. This routine procedure, performed under local anesthesia, can be done once and eliminate a lifetime of repeat visits to the podiatrist. It is also recommended for those who have a chronic, painful condition which has not been responsive to home and professional care.

Treatment

The first step in any treatment is to establish the cause of the corn. Is it the shoe, the underlying bone, or both?

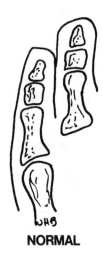 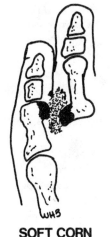

NORMAL   **SOFT CORN**
                        with bone deformity

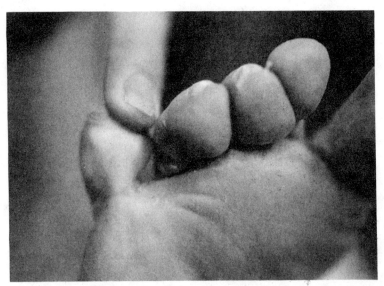

Soft corn located between the last two toes.

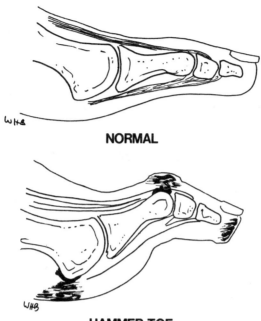

NORMAL

HAMMER TOE
contracted toe deformity

Improperly fitting shoes can cause corns. If you notice that your corn(s) only hurts in a particular shoe or shoe style, simply change your shoe style or—second best—have the shoes mechanically stretched by your local shoe repairman.

If your corn hurts in most shoes, your problem may be a hammertoe or underlying bone spur. Hammertoes are a deformity of the toe bones in which the "knuckle" of the toe rises above its normal position. This is caused by an imbalance of the muscles inserting into your toes. High-heel shoes can magnify this imbalance by providing the muscles inserting into the bottom of your toes with a mechanical advantage over the muscles which insert into the top. The result is that your toe "buckles up" under the pressure. The tendons on the top of your foot and toes then shorten. A hammertoe, being higher than a straight toe, is more apt to rub the top of your shoe. This rubbing is what produces the corn.

Bone spurs are actually bony growths which develop on the bones within your foot. They are made up of calcium, which is deposited by your body in response to increased pressure on a bone. In the same way that increased pressure causes the skin on the outside to grow, so will this pressure cause the underlying bone to grow. This calcium deposition is *not* directly linked to your dietary or metabolic utilization of the mineral calcium.

The best way to determine the cause of the problem is to have an X-ray taken of your foot. A bone spur or hammertoe is readily identifiable. If there is still a doubt as to etiology, it may be useful to have X-rays taken with and without shoes, to demonstrate how your feet respond to shoe pressure.

Years ago, before an adequate surgical cure was available, treatment of a chronic corn consisted of periodic cutting of the buildup of hard skin followed by the application of a small protective pad. If done improperly at home, this can be dangerous! Many infections and even loss of toes have resulted from this type of "bathroom" surgery. Conservative treatment is best left to a podiatrist who has both the experience and the sterile instruments to safely and effectively remove a corn.

Home Treatment

Do not attempt self-treatment if you suffer from any of the following conditions:

Diabetes
A foot infection
Poor circulation
An unsteady hand
Poor vision

Though home treatment is generally not recommended, here are some guidelines and precautions should you elect this course:

1. Be sure to perform removal in as sterile an environment as possible. Your feet should be soaked and cleaned thoroughly. If you are using a blade (*not recommended*), make sure it has been sterilized with seventy percent isopropyl alcohol before use.

2. *Never* apply over-the-counter corn medications such as Freezone®. These products are essentially acids. The acid cannot distinguish normal healthy skin from corns and calluses. Podiatrists routinely treat patients who have developed ulcers on the feet from such products.

3. If your corn worsens or simply does not improve, see a podiatrist.

Technique

Podiatrists Myles Schneider and Mark Sussman provide a good regimen for corn removal in their book *How to Doctor Your Feet Without the Doctor*:

1. Soak your feet for ten minues in one half gallon of warm water into which two tablespoons of household detergent has been added.

2. Dry the foot and rub a few drops of cooking oil into the corn to further soften it.

3. Use a pumice stone, sandpaper, or a callus file to gently remove the thickened skin. Use a back and forth sawing motion. Stop at the point where the skin begins to look normal.

4. Cover the corn with a one-eighth-inch *non-medicated* felt pad positioned so that the *hole* in the center of the pad is directly over the corn.

Calluses

Calluses are generally found over diffuse areas on the sole of the foot. Most often a buildup of callus will result in a "burning" sensation which will hurt more as the day progresses.

A variant of the callus is a painful localized lesion which occurs under a specific metatarsal on the ball of your foot. This condition, known as an intractable plantar keratoma (IPK) occurs when one or more metatarsals is lower than all the others.

Prevention

Calluses are more difficult to prevent than corns are because they are less dependent on the shoe you wear and more dependent on your foot structure and the way you walk.

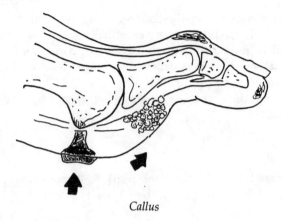

Callus

One way of reducing generalized callus is to wear anti-shearing insoles in your shoes. Two of the best available are Spenco (nitrogen impregnated foam) and PPT (a porometric material). These products are superior to the ordinary "foam" insoles which are commonly sold in drugstores and supermarkets. Ordinary foam insoles tend to be flimsy, deteriorate rapidly and are relatively ineffective in preventing the frictional shearing force responsible for most calluses.

For specific calluses, particularly IPK's, orthotic devices are the best prevention. Orthotics are custom shoe inserts, which resemble arch supports. Depressions can be built into an orthotic below the area of your callus. These depressions provide

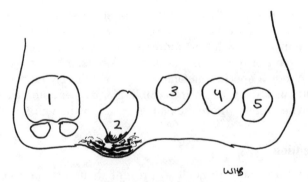

Intractable plantar keratoma (IPK)

space for the dropped bone (usually a metatarsal) to fit in. This prevents your bone from hitting the ground harder than the adjacent bones.

Orthotics will not correct the underlying structural condition which caused your callus. They will, however, provide accommodative relief. Correction of chronic calluses (particularly IPK's) may require metatarsal surgery (see Chapter Eleven).

Treatment

The treatment of calluses is essentially the same as the treatment of corns. Do not, however, try home treatment for an IPK—since these corn-like lesions are located deep in the sole, their safe removal requires the dexterity and equipment of a professional.

Heel Fissures

Heel fissures are painful cracks which form at the back or sides of your heel. These fissures are sometimes associated with callus formation and are found most often in heavy individuals and those who wear backless shoes.

Heel fissures are a potentially dangerous condition. One of the skin's primary functions is to protect the body from outside bacteria and open fissures of the skin allow these bacteria to enter and cause a heel infection. Because the skin at the back of the heel has a very poor vascular supply, your body will have difficulty healing such an infection.

Prevention

If you suffer from chronic heel fissures:

1. Wear closed back shoes whenever possible. Even sandals can be bought with a closed back.

2. Develop a regular foot care regimen. Each night soak your feet for twenty minutes in warm water to which an oil such as Alpha Keri® has been added. Pat dry and apply a moisturizing cream or ointment. Wrap the heel in Saran Wrap® and cover with a sock.

3. Don't let yourself become overweight.

4. If you begin to form a fissure, apply some tincture of benzoin to the heel area. This is an over-the-counter medication which forms a protective film to seal out bacteria and help prevent friction.

Treatment

Treatment is directed at prevention of an infection. The overlying callus should first be removed (see section on self-treatment of a corn). Apply a disinfectant such as alcohol or Betadine® to the fissure. Next apply a topical antibiotic ointment and cover with dry sterile gauze. If the condition fails to improve or if the heel becomes red, hot, or if you notice pus, see a podiatrist or physician.

Athlete's Foot

This common and annoying condition of the skin and nails is actually a fungal infection. Itching, scaling, redness, and even the formation of small blisters can occur, depending on which species you contract. Usually the web spaces (particularly between the fourth and fifth toes) become involved, resulting in painful fissures. Fungus can even affect your nails, causing them to become thickened and discolored.

Athlete's foot is also known as *tinea pedis* and "ringworm." The term "athlete's foot" came about for advertising reasons. In her book *On Your Feet*, Dr. Elizabeth Roberts relates a story she was told some years ago by a member of a public relations firm who had attended a conference promoting an over-the-counter antifungal medication: "Sales had been dropping. The group decided on a sales campaign in which the condition would be called policeman's foot. A few months after the launching of the campaign, another conference was called. The sales had plummeted so badly that the agency feared the loss of the account. The conclusion of the group was that too few people wanted to be associated with policemen! Then some bright soul suggested that everybody enjoyed being thought of as an athlete, so why not call it athlete's foot? And thus was born the term that has permeated lay literature and saved one account for a determined agency."

Athletes do suffer from this condition. So can you, if you create a skin environment conducive for fungi to thrive on. Fungi are plantlike organisms (some are related to the common mushroom). Fungal infections themselves present little danger to the body, because they do not, as a rule, enter the bloodstream. They can, however, mechanically bore small holes in the skin, which allow bacteria to enter. Fungal infections are contagious and should be treated, especially in the case of systemic diseases such as diabetes.

Fungi like to live in a warm, moist, dark environment. A shoe provides such an environment. Fungi are everywhere, so the best way to prevent them from infecting your foot is to establish a shoe climate least suitable for their growth:

1. Choose a shoe made of natural materials. Natural materials such as leather and canvas allow this moisture to escape and let the foot "breathe."

2. Apply a little cornstarch to your shoes before and after wearing them. Cornstarch is more absorbent than talc and contains fewer impurities.

3. Keep your shoes dry. Do not wear them on consecutive days. It takes two to three days for a shoe to adequately dry out. One way you can accelerate this process is to use your hair dryer for a few minutes at a medium heat setting. Another method is to stuff your shoes with old newspapers. Leaving your shoes near a heater is less desirable because it may cause the leather of the shoe to shrink.

4. Clean your feet thoroughly at least twice a day. Fungi are parasites which survive by "eating" the outside layer of your dead skin. Soap and water help to remove this layer. Be sure to thoroughly dry your feet afterward, paying particular attention to the web spaces in between your toes.

5. Change your socks at least twice a day. If your feet tend to sweat, select stockings with a high cotton content. Cotton serves to "wick" moisture to the surface which helps keep the feet cool and dry.

6. If you have a tendency toward fungal infections, apply an over-the-counter powder such as Tinactin® daily to your shoes and socks.

Treatment

The first step in the treatment of fungal infections is to establish a diagnosis and determine which specific organism is causing your problems. Athlete's foot must be differentiated from other skin conditions such as allergic shoe dermatitis, erythrasma, and even syphilis.

Your podiatrist or physician will take a small sample of infected skin or nail. He can then grow this organism in a culture medium. In a week or two, the particular species can be identified.

Topical Medications

Clotrimazole, which is a prescription medication marketed under the names Lotrimin® and Mycelex® is the most effective broad spectrum antifungal drug available today. It comes as a cream or solution and is far more effective than are over-the-counter products such as Tinactin® and Desenex®.

Oral Antifungals

If your infection does not respond to topical medications, you may require an oral antifungal. Griseofulvin is the most widely used and safest of these. Nizoral® (ketocanizole) is a newer, more powerful medication, reserved for severe fungal infections. Nizoral is contraindicated for those who have impaired liver function.

Fungal Nails

Thickened or discolored nails generally result from fungal infections. Fungi work their way under the nail, which provides a near perfect "greenhouse" for them. Fungi thrive under nails and gradually consume the nail, rotting it in the process. Sometimes a fungal nail may completely separate from the underlying skin and may even fall off completely.

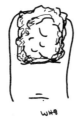

MYCOTIC NAIL INFECTION
fungous

Treatment

Fungal nails are a frustrating condition to treat. Topical antifungal medications are not effective in the treatment of badly infected nails and even oral antifungals are of limited value. They must be used for many months and after you stop using them, the fungus may return.

For many people, the only effective treatment may be the total removal of the infected nail. Regardless of which treatment is used, the most important element is persistence. Once a fungus entrenches itself in your nails, it is only by following a stringent treatment program that you can fully and permanently rid yourself of this condition.

Plantar Warts

These are benign growths found on the bottom (plantar) surface of the foot and are also known as verrucae or papillomas. Warts are not caused by toads. They are actually small external tumors caused by a papilloma virus.

Warts are initially contracted by stepping on a wet abrasive virus-infested surface (hence the connection with toads) such as the concrete surrounding a swimming pool or the bottom surface of a shower. Abrasion acts to rub the virus particles into the sole of your foot. This explains why warts generally occur on the weight-bearing surfaces of your foot such as under the metatarsals or on the heel. Because warts develop in areas where normal callus would form, it is often difficult to tell the difference between the two. Warts are sometimes covered with a layer of callus, which must first be removed to establish the diagnosis.

Once the overlying callus has been removed, a wart with the following characteristics will be revealed:

1. It will be round and have a discrete border. This border is often described as a "moat."

2. The skin will be pinkish-white and a different shade than the yellow tint of a corn or callus (similar to fingerprints).

3. There will be an absence of skin lines within the wart. These lines resemble fingerprints.

4. Small red dots may be seen within the wart. These are small capillaries feeding the tumor. When a wart is trimmed, it will bleed, while a corn or callus will not.

Plantar warts are slow-growing and may take several months to become large enough to cause pain. If you notice a suspicious growth on your foot, be sure to have it checked out as soon as possible. The larger you let the wart grow, the more difficult it will become to treat. Warts left untreated can spread to other parts of your foot and may even spread to your hands.

Prevention

The virus that causes warts likes to live in the same warm, moist, dark environment as the fungus. So, the same general steps you would take to prevent a fungal infection (keeping your foot dry) will also help prevent warts. Additionally, you should wear thongs or protective shoes whenever you are in a situation conducive to viral contact.

Wart viruses are present near swimming pools, shower stalls, and at the beach. Most papilloma viruses are picked up during the summer, when you're most likely to go barefoot. This explains the abundance of wart infected feet which show up in podiatrists's offices during the early fall (after they have grown large enough to become painful).

Wearing a pair of thongs or jellies (rubber shoes for children) is the most effective way of preventing a wart infection. Children seem to be highly receptive to verrucae. As you get older, your chances of getting a wart seem to decrease. It has not been determined whether this is because older people spend less time barefoot or whether immunological factors are involved.

There are also psychological factors involved in the treatment of warts. Young children seem to respond well to placebo medications. Recently a four-year-old was brought into my office with multiple warts on his left foot. I told the boy that I was applying a "magic medicine" to his warts which would make them disappear within three weeks. When he returned a month later, his warts were gone. Only the boy's mother and I knew that this "magic" medicine was clear nail polish.

Treatment

The earlier the treatment, the more effective the cure. If a wart is diagnosed early enough, it may respond to an over-the-counter medication such as Compound W®. Products of this sort contain a mild acid which destroys wart tissue. If you decide to use such a product, have a doctor first confirm the diagnosis. Many times people think they have a wart when they have a corn, callus, or even skin cancer (malignant melanoma). It's one thing to attempt self-treatment and quite another to attempt self-diagnosis!

Podiatrists and dermatologists can offer a wide array of alternative treatments, among them dry ice, electro-dessication, vitamin A injections, surgical curettage, strong acid treatments, and laser ablation. Hundreds of additional treatments have been tried, including the injection of wart tissue back into the body, anti-cancer drugs and even hypnosis, but no one method has emerged as being totally effective.

Advocates of each therapy claim high or even complete success rates, but controlled studies of a large enough sample eventually disprove such claims. Most verruca specialists acknowledge a recurrence rate of five to fifteen percent even with the most effective treatments.

Your doctor's choice of treatment will depend on his preference and on the size and number of warts you have. The amount of time you are willing to spend to get rid of your warts may also be a factor in the treatment selection.

If you have a large number of small lesions (sometimes referred to as "mosaic" warts), he may elect for the periodic application of a strong acid, such as forty percent salicylic acid or mono-, bi-, or trichlorocetic acid. This process may require many repeat visits to his office and is somewhat tedious, but is less traumatic than other methods.

If you have a solitary lesion, he may elect to use curettage (under local anesthesia) to remove the entire verruca in one visit. In this technique a surgical curette is used to "scoop" the entire wart out. An acid such as phenol is then applied to the base of the wart to help prevent its recurrence. Many busy people prefer this method to the long, drawn out acid treatments.

Every few years a new "miracle" treatment evolves for the treatment of warts. The use of the surgical laser is one of the latest of these fads. A laser generates a powerful concentrated beam of light which literally vaporizes the wart. Laser surgery is less traumatic than conventional surgical curettage because the laser anesthesizes the local nerves as it vaporizes tissue.

Erythrasma

Redness between the toes can occasionally be due to erythrasma, a condition which mimics athlete's feet. This skin infection is caused by the parasitic organism cornyebacterium, which is classified as being between a bacteria and a fungi. Erythrasma does not respond to antifungal medications and is often misdiagnosed. Erythrasma infected skin fluoresces green when illuminated by a Wood's light, which is the best method of confirming a diagnosis. Erthyrasma infections respond well to the oral antibiotic erythromycin.

Dermatitis

Dermatitis is a generalized term for many skin conditions which cause irritation to your skin. This irritation can cause your skin to become red, itchy, and even painful. Often small blisters referred to as bullae can form.

Dermatitis can be caused by direct contact with a caustic substance (such as an acid), or by exposure to an allergic compound (such as a dye, glue or tanning compound found in your shoe).

Many cosmetics and nail products contain allergic compounds. Dermatitis can even occur on your feet as a result of an internal medicine or food. Another form of this condition is known as neurodermatitis and is the result of constant itching of the skin, stemming from a psychological or neurological problem.

Treatment of dermatitis should first be directed at finding and eliminating the underlying cause of the disorder. If dermatitis is present as a result of allergy to a substance found in a particular shoe, patch testing should be done to isolate the offending substance. Often special hypo-allergenic shoes must be ordered (see Chapter Two). If the dermatitis can be traced to a specific medication, food or cosmetic product, this substance should likewise be avoided.

Neurodermatitis often responds to psychological treatments and anti-anxiety medications such as tranquilizers. Atarax® is an effective medication for use in this condition because it has both a tranquilizer and an antihistamine action.

When the cause of foot dermatitis cannot be positively ascertained or controlled, symptomatic treatment should be used. Strong soaps or detergents should not be used to wash the irritated skin of the foot. Avenno Bar® and Lowila Cake® are gentle hypo-allergenic products which can be used to cleanse the skin. Topical steroid creams are effective in relieving the redness and itching associated with dermatitis. Steroids are derivatives of cortisone, a natural anti-inflammatory produced in your adrenal glands. Mild over-the-counter preparations are available (such as .5% hydrocortisone) and may be of value. If your condition does not respond to this medication, see your podiatrist or dermatologist. It may be necessary for him to prescribe a topical steroid.

Nails

Toenails serve very little useful purpose. You can do very well without them. This was not so for primitive man whose toenails were of great assistance in helping him to climb trees.

For the modern shoe wearer, nails are just another foot part to take care of, to be cut properly, and perhaps to be covered with polish.

Your toenails are made up of keratin, a modified skin protein

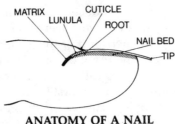

ANATOMY OF A NAIL

very much related to your hair. Most of the visible nail is actually dead, the only live part being the nail root, which lies under the cuticle.

Contrary to popular belief, nails do not grow after you are dead. This misconception is based on the fact that the skin and cuticles around the nail shrink rapidly after death, creating the illusion that the nails are still growing. Nails *are* extremely slow growing, taking about six months to fully replace themselves. There is very little you can do to alter the rate of growth or shape of the nail. Scientific research has disproved the popular myth that the ingestion of gelatin can speed the growth of nails.

The condition of your nails can often reflect your systemic health. Circulatory diseases such as arteriosclerosis and chronic respiratory conditions such as tuberculosis and lung cancer exhibit noticeable changes in the nails.

Beau's lines are transverse ridges in the nail which document systemic disease in the same way that the rings in a tree stump tell of the life of the tree. Beau's lines result from an interruption of the growth plate of the nail, known as the matrix. Severe systemic diseases ranging from diabetes to psoriasis can cause these lines to appear.

Thickened Toenails

Generalized thickening or clubbing of the nails sometimes results from chronic respiratory conditions such as tuberculosis or lung cancer. When only one or two nails are thickened, it is usually the result of localized trauma. If someone steps on your toe or if you drop a heavy object on your toe, there's a good chance that the new nail which grows in will be thicker than the

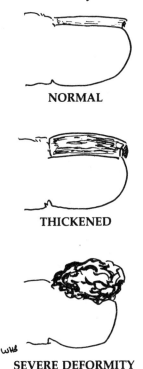

NORMAL

THICKENED

SEVERE DEFORMITY

original nail. Treatment of such nails usually consists of periodic grinding of the nail to decrease its thickness. In cases where shoe fitting is a problem, it is sometimes best to permanently remove the nail. Usually a callused skin develops where the nail once was. This resembles the nail and can be covered with polish. As was mentioned previously, toenails have little function and you can do very well without them.

Ingrown Toenails

The most common and most painful nail condition is the ingrown toenail. This occurs when the side of the nail cuts into the surrounding skin. Improper cutting of the nails is generally responsible for this malady, with tight and improperly fitting shoes an aggravating factor.

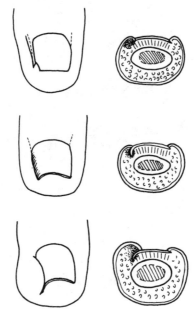

Three stages of an ingrown toenail (from The Foot Book*)*

Prevention

Adequate length and proper cutting of toenails will prevent ingrowing from occuring. Nail length should extend slightly farther than the end of the toe. Cutting your nails too short may precipitate an ingrown nail.

Trimming should be done with a good nail clipper. Many ingrown nails result from the "picking" or ripping of nails. This habit is particularly common in children and teenagers. Often a small piece known as a "spicule" is left which can easily grow into the adjacent skin. Never cut into the corners of your nails. This practice can also lead to spicule formation.

The proper method of cutting a toenail is straight across. Most nails are not flat. It is usually best to follow the natural slope of the nail when cutting across. It is often advisable to make several small cuts instead of one large one. A nail file or emery board should be used to finish off the nail.

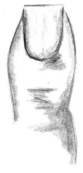 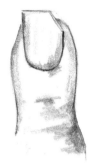 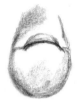

Proper way   *Improper way*   *Follow the contour*
to cut the nail   *to cut the nail*   *of the nail*

Treatment

If you sense a toenail is beginning to ingrow, it may be possible to treat it yourself. Soak your feet in some lukewarm water to soften up the nail. Take a small wisp of cotton (such as from the end of a Q-tip® and gently place it into the sulcus between the nail edge and the adjoining skin. Leave the cotton in for a few weeks. *Do not* cut a "V" into the center of the nail. This is a folk remedy that mistakenly assumed that the nail will be forced to grow toward the center and thus away from the ingrown edge. It is a gross misconception! All nails grow in only one direction—from back to front.

One over-the-counter remedy which may be helpful is Outgro®, which contains tannic acid. This serves to toughen the skin on the side of the nail and resist ingrowing. While these home remedies may be helpful for mild ingrown nails, professional help is necessary for more severe cases.

Nail Infections

Nail infections often result from inadequate home treatment of ingrown toenails. Typically a patient comes in after "battling" an ingrown nail for many weeks. Usually the history goes something like this: "After I soak the foot, the toe feels better. Then a few hours later it hurts again. I saw some pus so I put some antibiotic cream on. It got a little better, but now it's worse again."

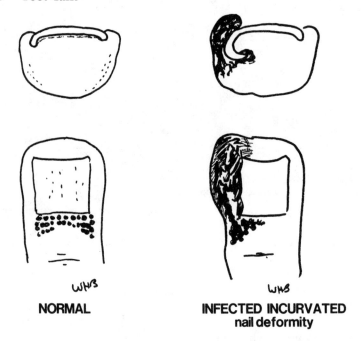

NORMAL

INFECTED INCURVATED
nail deformity

What the patient doesn't realize is that the infection can only be resolved if the offending nail spicule is removed. If the infection is allowed to progress, the skin surrounding the nail becomes chronically infected. This condition is known as pyogenic granuloma or "proud flesh" and is characterized by swelling, pain and frequent bleeding. Pyogenic granuloma requires surgical intervention and appropriate use of an antibiotic.

Nail Surgery

If you suffer from chronic ingrown nails, a relatively simple and painless corrective procedure is available. Under local anesthesia, a small section of the ingrown side of a nail is removed. A chemical acid (phenol) is then applied to the nail root and matrix to prevent its regrowth. This procedure is non-disabling and highly effective.

The Foot Beautiful   4

Beautiful feet have been the aspiration of women since the beginning of recorded time. Ancient history's most famous beautician—who also deserves the title "mother of podiatry"—was Cleopatra, Queen of the Nile. In ancient times, podiatry was an integral part of cosmetology, the science of creating and preserving the beauty of the human body. Cleopatra wrote a textbook on cosmetics, which, though lost, has been passed on to us at least in partial form via the famous physician Galenos, who copied some of the chapters. Cleopatra divided cosmetics into podiatry (care of the feet and pedicuring), chiriatry (care of the hands and manicuring), dermatiatry (skin care), komiatry (hair care), and odontiatry (care of the teeth).

Keeping your feet looking beautiful requires only a few minutes a day, and the efforts are well worth it. Beautiful feet feel better and are healthier for the rest of you. If you neglect them, you may develop overly dry or excessively sweaty skin. Neglected feet can also develop a notorious foul smell. These problems can all be prevented or minimized with the proper beauty regimen.

Sweaty Feet

Because the feet are among the hardest-working parts of the body, they normally perspire heavily. The average pair of feet sweat at least one full cup of fluid daily. The feet contain a large number of sweat glands. When you walk or run, these glands secrete fluid. These glands are also activated when your feet get hot. Evaporation of sweat serves to cool them off.

Nervousness also triggers perpiration in the soles. This occurs simultaneously with the sweating of the palms experienced during periods of stress or anxiety. If you tend to be "high strung" your feet will perspire excessively.

Prevention

Prevention of sweaty feet is directed at allowing accumulated perspiration to evaporate. Wearing "breathable" shoes and socks of natural materials will help, as well as selecting shoes with an upper made of a natural material such as leather or canvas. Avoid man-made materials like vinyl. Cotton (warm weather) and wool (cold weather) are superior to nylon, orlon, or other synthetics. In general, natural fibers act to "wick" excess moisture away from the skin.

Try to change your shoes and socks as often as possible during the day. Many women use a walking shoe or sneaker to get to work and then change into a more fashionable shoe. This serves many functions, not the least of which is to better distribute moisture. For this reason it is a good idea not to wear the same pair of shoes on two consecutive days.

As mentioned, adding cornstarch to your shoes and socks (more absorbent than talc and less expensive) is helpful in preventing the accumulation of moisture. Cornstarch is available in your local grocery or supermarket and scented varieties can be purchased in your pharmacy.

Antiperspirants can also help prevent sweaty feet. You may use conventional spray-on or roll-on products or for better value, ask your pharmacist for a bottle of twenty-five percent aluminum chloride tincture. Aluminum chloride is the active ingredient in most antiperspirants and is thought to decrease the amount of fluid secreted by changing the polarity of the sweat glands.

If all of the above measures do not resolve your problem, see your podiatrist or dermatologist. He may prescribe appropriate oral medications.

Foot Odor

This condition is technically known as bromhidrosis and is caused by an accumulation of bacteria, fungus, mold, and yeast on your feet. Foot odor is compounded by the rotting of the materials within your shoes caused by the caustic action of your perspiration.

Bromhidrosis can also be caused by the ingestion of aromatic foods and spices. A woman patient complained of periodic bouts of foot odor. After a careful history it became evident that these incidents correlated to her use of garlic in cooking. When she stopped using garlic, her problem disappeared.

Foot odor is socially unacceptable. It connotes bad hygiene. Prevention is directed at keeping the feet both clean and dry. In his book *Dr. Zismor's Skin Care Book*, Jonathan Zismor recommends a good antideodorant soap such as Safeguard® or Palmolive Gold®, but he cautions that these soaps may cause photosensitization of the skin and predispose you to a bad sunburn.

Washing your feet with a small amount of Betadine® (povidine iodine) scrub is the most effective method of killing surface bacteria. pHisoHex® is also effective, but requires a doctor's prescription.

Over-the-counter insoles are generally of little value in controlling bromhidrosis. If your problem does not respond to the aforementioned suggestions, see your podiatrist or dermatologist.

Dry Skin

Your skin is lubricated by sebaceous (oil containing) glands. As you get older, these glands become less active and your skin is likely to become dryer.

Excessive washing of the skin will also cause dryness. Caustic soaps and detergents in particular deplete the skin of its natural oils.

Dry skin gives you the appearance of being older than you are. This accounts for the tremendous sales success of moisturizing creams and lotions. But you must remember that moisturizers do not add moisture to your skin. They merely act to prevent moisture from escaping. In fact, the most potent moisturizing agent known to man is also the most common: plain tap water. Soaking your feet in water is the best way to add moisture to your skin. But be careful—excessive washing of the feet will actually dry out the skin because it strips your body of its natural oils. For value, you can't beat plain vegetable shortening such as Crisco® to seal that moisture in—it's just as good as the expensive moisturizers in the fancy bottles.

There is a proper way to use the various products available. Alpha-Keri creme®, Nivea®, Vaseline Intensive Care Lotion®, and Jergens Hand Creme® are all good. First soak your feet for a few minutes in warm water. This hydrates (adds water to) the skin. It's a good idea to add some bath oil such as Alpha-Keri® to the water. Then pat the feet dry. The only part of the feet that should be thoroughly dried is between the toes (this area is naturally moist). Next apply a liberal amount of your moisturizing creme or lotion. For maximum efficiency, place a layer of food wrap such as Saran Wrap® over the foot and cover with a sock. This effectively seals in moisture.

Beautiful Nails

Beautiful nails enhance the foot. For the proper way to cut your nails see the nail section of Chapter Three.

Pedicuring is the phase of cosmetology dealing with nail care. Done properly, pedicuring is a safe and effective method of keeping your nails looking their best.

Be careful when you push back the nail's cuticle. The cuticle protects the nail root and matrix and when it is pushed back too far, bacteria can enter and cause an infection known as a paronychia (par-o-nick'-ea).

Nail polish is not only decorative but also helps prevent the nail from chipping or cracking. Clear polish is adequate for normal wear. Colored polishes add a special glamor to your feet. Regardless of which you choose, be sure to first make certain that you are not allergic to any of the ingredients in the polish. If you're using a new brand or color, place a small amount on one nail one day before you polish all your nails. If you have no reaction, it is safe to continue using that color. Hypoallergenic polishes are available from several manufacturers.

Allergic reactions may also result from the use of artificial nails. It's usually the glues used to attach the artificial nail that are responsible for this reaction.

Artificial nails are most useful in cases where a toenail has been damaged or surgically removed.

Ten Minutes a Day to More Beautiful Feet

Beautiful feet are possible!!! But you'll have to give them the same type of attention you give your hair, hands, and face. Get into a daily regimen and your feet will look and feel better.

1. Start by soaking your feet in warm water for about five minutes. You may do this in your bath or in a separate tub. If your skin is dry add some bath oil to the water. Use of a soap which contains lanolin or cold cream such as Dove® or Caress® or a superfatted soap like Basis®, will also be helpful. Oily skin responds will to a drying soap such as Fostex® or Ivory®. If your skin is normal add some Johnson's Foot Soap® to the water.

2. Use a Buf-puf®, Loofa®, or Tawashi® to gently remove the outer layer of dead skin from your feet. If you have a moderate amount of callus, use a pumice stone with a similar motion.

3. Pat your feet dry. The only area of the feet you need dry thoroughly is between your toes. Apply a liberal coat of moisturizing creme to the feet (except between the toes). If your skin is particularly dry, cover with Saran Wrap and encase in a stocking. If the skin on your heels is rough, use an abrasive creme such as Pretty Feet®.

4. At the end of your beauty regimen elevate your feet—all day long they're working. Give them a rest!

The Erotic Foot 5

The visual sensuality of the foot's contours, convolutions and toe cleavage make it an organ of erotic association. In addition, the foot is one of the most innervated parts of the body, containing thousands of tiny, yet sensitive receptors. These terminals supply the brain not only with pain and temperature information (like the skin elsewhere on the body) but with a sense of pressure and body position. These nerve endings account for the foot's sensitivity which often takes the form of ticklishness.

In his classic work, *The Sex Life of the Foot and Shoe*, William Rossi says:

> The human foot possesses a natural sexuality whose powers have borne remarkable influence on all peoples of all cultures throughout all history . . . The shoe is no simple, protective housing for the foot, nor a whimsical decoration. It serves chiefly as a sexual covering for the foot's natural erotic character. Footwear fashion is podoerotic art.

Fetishes involving the foot and shoe, also known as equus eroticus, are the most common of sexual novelties. Rossi quotes from a popular fetish magazine publisher:

> When we started our magazine on sex fetishes, we expected to cover the whole range. But our mail and other

feedback quickly told us that the foot and shoe fetishists outnumbered any other fetish group by at least three to one.

In his *Studies in the Psychology of Sex*, Havelock Ellis states, "Of all the forms of erotic symbolism, the most frequent is that which idealizes the foot and shoe."

Look around. Obvious signs of sexual emphasis are everywhere . . . just one example is the shiny, brightly colored openbacked heeled shoe. Often the front of the shoe is cut open, revealing protruding toes and foot cleavage.

Freud declares the shoe or slipper a "symbol of the female genitals." The shoe has always been associated with fertility customs, marriage and romance.

Many of us can remember from elementary school hearing about the gallant Sir Walter Raleigh spreading his cape over a muddied street so that Queen Elizabeth could cross without dirtying her slippers.

The drinking of wine from the dainty slipper of a lover is a well-known symbol of romance. Many a lover has attested to the attributes of this ambrosia.

The custom of tying shoes to the departing car of newlyweds is symbolic of the sexual union and there are countless versions of this custom being played out in different cultures.

The foot itself is responsible, says Rossi, for the erotic image of the entire human body. Upright posture and bipedal gait created the figure as we know it, bringing bosom, abdomen and thighs into view. It created erogenous zones and visual sex appeal features. This position made human frontal copulation, unique in all nature, possible. Visual stimuli and continuity of sexual excitement led to year-round sex. This was the beginning of our psychosexual inhibitions and fantasies.

Freud discusses how the role of scent as a sexual stimulant in animals and insects was replaced by visual stimuli in humans.

It is our bipedal stance that literally lifted us from the ground, exposed us, leading to feelings of shame and modesty. Therefore we have an innate sense that the feet are somehow responsible for our sexuality.

Florenz Ziegfeld, whose beautiful showgirls graced the stages of the 1920s, interviewed the girls by first watching them walk in high heels from behind a white screen, thus seeing only their silhouettes. "Before I see their faces, I want to see how they walk. There's more sex in a walk than in a face or even in a figure."

Gypsy Rose Lee, the famous stripper, knew the power of a high-heeled shoe. This great sexual teaser would never be caught on stage without a magnificent pair of shoes.

The high heel and the position it creates for the foot is a strong sexual stimulus. The feet are plantar-flexed (not perpendicular to the leg as they are in a relaxed position). This is the position emphasized for the foot in any centerfold picture. It is also achieved in the sexy crossing of legs where one foot teasingly flexes forward. The extension of the foot, pointing of the toes, particularly with a circular movement, is a strong body language signal saying "I'm available."

In women another attribute of sexuality is small feet. The tiny delicate foot is extolled in the shoe store as it is in literature. The Cinderella story promotes the virtues of the small foot as a symbol of feminity and sexual desirability. With hundreds of versions throughout the world this folk tale often bordered on erotic literature. It was the Grimm brothers who tamed it for children.

One of the oldest known versions dates back to ancient Egypt where a beautiful girl named Rhodopis was bathing in the River Nile when an eagle swooped down and flew off to Memphis with one of her dainty slippers. This he deposited at the foot of King Psamtik. The king was overcome with passion for the owner of the slipper. He envisioned her image with lecherous eagerness. Obsessed by thoughts of the girl, he journeyed through the kingdom, trying the slipper on the feet of young maidens until he finally found Rhodopis and married her. The Third Pyramid of Gizeh stands as testimony to this union.

In seventeenth-century Europe, Perrault wrote another version of the Cinderella story with obvious erotic inferences, many of which were lost in the translation from French. Rossi states that his image of the foot being inserted into a furry slipper has phallic-yoni symbolism. "The romantic union of the prince and Cinderella was sexually symbolized by the suggestive union of the virginal phallic foot and the furry yoni shoe."

A ninth-century Chinese version of the Cinderella tale, Rossi suggests, may have given rise to the custom of footbinding which exemplifies the ultimate in foot eroticism and fetish.

For nearly one thousand years this podoerotomania captivated the Chinese imagination. The foot took on a new role in human sexuality, becoming a sexual organ itself. Hundreds of millions of people were caught up in this sexual mania, the lingering effects of which can even be seen today in the feet of some elderly Chinese women. Even non-Orientals living in China were devotees of the practice. "Unbound women" were stigmatized with remarks such as "goosefoot" and "demon with huge feet."

Chinese males were obsessed with the sexuality of the bound foot, dreaming of catching a glimpse of the desirable appendage unfettered. The "lotus foot" as it was called (because the resulting walk resembled the delicate swaying movement of the lotus plant in the wind) was regarded as the most erotic part of the entire female anatomy. Pornography and prostitution centered around the lotus foot. Intellectuals, warriors and noblemen were as charmed by its aphrodisiac powers as were the common folk. Religious movements were completely ineffective in trying to stop the licentious foot-binding practice.

The Chinese always had a fascination for small feet, regarding them as a sign of fine breeding and grace. They scaled down the foot to accommodate this image, often to a mere four inches long.

The process was begun in girls of five or six years of age, when their bones were soft and malleable. The four small toes were bent under the ball of the foot as far as possible and secured with progressively tighter bandages. The large toe was left free for propulsion in walking, and for balance. The foot was gradually bent as a cross bow, bringing heel and toes as close together as possible. The heel bone was brought into a near vertical position and a high arch was created.

The bandages served in much the same manner as a brace does for the teeth, redirecting growth and shaping to the desired effect. There was a great deal of discomfort from the bandages but girls grew immune to it much in the same way that women today have accommodated pointed shoes and high heels. In fact, upon X-ray the lotus foot resembles the X-ray foot of a woman in high heels.

The normal hard callus tissue on the bottom of the foot became soft and fleshy in the deep cleft of the arch. Chinese men found the way these women walked—on the tops of their toes in a delicate, willowy gait—extremely exciting.

Because of the great difficulty the women had in walking they were excluded from the drudgery of hard work. Imagine women working in a corn field in extremely high heeled shoes!

It seems that women have always been amenable to having their feet deformed, thereby altering their gait and creating the illusion of tiny feet.

Rossi said, "If the Chinese concentrated their deformation on the foot, American, European, and other women (and often men) have for centuries been doing the same with tight shoes, the wearing of styles that have no kinship with natural foot shape, high heels that force alterations in the whole anatomy, stiff-soled shoes that prevent natural foot function, laced shoes and boots that impede circulation, and platform soles that can jeopardize human life itself."

Yet women continue to get pleasure from wearing shoes that intoxicate the male psyche. They endure the pain for the satisfaction of being more sexually desirable.

The women's liberation movement initially made inroads into this self-inflicted podomasochism and for a while more sensible low heeled styles were in fashion. Even comfortable sports shoes were worn on the job. These, however, have been in direct conflict with the erotic nature of the foot.

The executive woman soon realized that she could do a man's job but she was not psychosexually comfortable walking in a man's shoes. So we are returning to the days where the shoes fit the psyche, not the foot.

The Walking Foot   6

Most people take walking for granted. What we fail to realize is that while it may be one of the most fundamental of all body functions, it is also one of the most complex. With each step, the foot must compensate for a multitude of factors, not the least of which is our often unpredictable terrain. Consider this: the foot enables you to walk 100,000 miles in your lifetime. Each foot contains 26 bones, 19 muscles and 107 ligaments. Leonardo da Vinci described the foot as "a masterpiece of engineering and a work of art."

How We Walk

Walking has often been described as a series of controlled falls in which you are continually falling forward only to catch yourself with the next step—just watch a young child as he learns to walk. But the momentum imparted by falling forward is actually just a small part of walking. To insure a smooth gait, dozens of muscles of the hips, thighs, legs, and feet must contract in precise sequence with each step. Weakness or injury in any of these muscles will hinder walking, often resulting in a limp. The structure of the entire skeleton also influences the way we walk. Do your feet point straight ahead when you walk or do they turn in or out? Look at your knees. Are you bowlegged or knock-kneed? These conditions are all determined by rotations and positions of your bones.

The Foot In Walking

The foot plays one of the most important roles in walking. It must compensate for every structural abnormality in the skeleton above. The foot must modify its function for such conditions as a curved spine (scoliosis), limb length difference, and muscle shortening or imbalance. The failure of the foot to adequately adapt to structural imperfections in the body will result in the eventual breakdown of foot structure. It is this collapse of the foot—known as *abnormal pronation*—which leads to flat feet, heel spurs, bunions and hammertoes and is also responsible for "runner's knee" (chondromalacia), as well as many cases of hip and back pain.

The Gait Cycle

To help you better understand how the foot functions (and malfunctions) during walking, let's examine the phases of just one step. The first part of the gait cycle is known as heel contact. This begins as the outside part of your heel touches the ground. If you examine the bottom of a well worn shoe, you'll notice that the outside part of the heel is worn more than the inside. This is normal. During this heel contact stage, your foot pronates, causing your foot bones to become loose. You may have noticed that I mentioned the term *abnormal pronation* before to describe a destructive force. This normal pronation is the same force but over a shorter period of time. The foot *must* pronate for a moment at heel contact to adapt to an often uneven walking surface. This initial pronation also acts as a shock absorber for the upper body and helps to smooth out the walking pattern. Abnormal pronation is a condition in which the foot continues to collapse beyond this initial phase.

The next phase of gait is known as *mid-stance*. At this point the leg is directly above the foot and the bones and joints of the foot should now be moving in the opposite direction of pronation. This motion is known as supination and causes the foot to act as a rigid lever. It is necessary for the foot to be rigid for the next stage of gait, which is known as the propulsive phase. In this stage, the leg passes over the foot and the heel lifts off. In individuals with short or tightened calf muscles, this heel lift may be premature and result in a "bopping" or jerky gait. This condition

One complete gait cycle of right limb

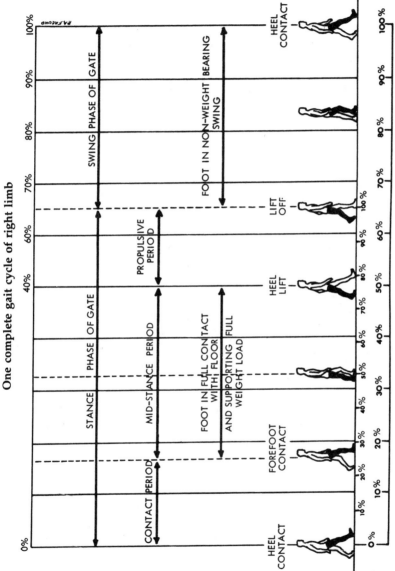

P.A.FAEUHR

SWING PHASE OF GATE

FOOT IN NON-WEIGHT BEARING SWING

HEEL CONTACT

PROPULSIVE PERIOD

LIFT OFF

STANCE   PHASE   OF GATE

MID-STANCE   PERIOD

HEEL LIFT

FOOT IN FULL CONTACT WITH FLOOR AND SUPPORTING FULL WEIGHT LOAD

FOREFOOT CONTACT

CONTACT PERIOD

HEEL CONTACT

0%   10%   20%   30%   40%   50%   60%   70%   80%   90%   100%

is known as *equinus* and derives its name because the foot structure resembles that of a horse's raised heel. Like pronation, equinus is a destructive force on the foot.

Propulsion is completed as we push off our toes. The big toe exerts the greatest force in this action, with a relatively insignificant contribution from each of the lesser toes.

The final stage of gait is known as the *swing* phase. During this period, your thigh flexes and your leg extends, swinging your foot forward where it prepares for the next step.

Arch Height

The structure of your foot also influences the way you walk. The height of your arch is an important structural feature. How high is yours? Remove your shoes and socks and examine your arch height. Next, take a step down and look at your arch again. Is it low, medium, or high? Did the height of your arch drop significantly when you put weight on it? Which arch height is best?

Keep in mind that the height of the arch does not indicate foot function. Both high and low arched feet can function well.

What happens to the height of the arch on weightbearing, is actually more important than the actual height of the arch itself. A dramatic decrease in the arch when you step down is a sign of abnormal pronation. This "collapsed foot" is known as a hypermobile flatfoot and is often referred to as "fallen arches." If you look closely at the inside borders of such feet you will often see what appears as two ankle bones. What you are actually seeing is the protruding head of a foot bone called the talus. Another sign of abnormal pronation are small blister-like sacs which can be seen on the inside edge of the heel. These outpouchings which occur only on weightbearing are known as "pronation blebs."

The abnormally pronated foot must be differentiated from the ordinary low arched foot. An arch which is low and remains the same both off and on weightbearing is probably perfectly normal. During World War I, U.S. Army medical officials mistakenly refused to accept soldiers with "flatfeet." Low arched feet (as opposed to abnormally pronated feet) are actually very sta-

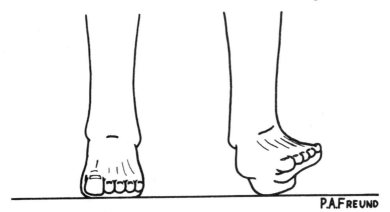

P.A.FREUND

IDEAL FOOT POSITION   PRONATED FOOT POSITION

ble—many of the National Football's League's premier linemen have them.

Most authorities, however, agree that a medium arch height is the most desirable. People with arches of medium height suffer less foot injury than either people with high or low arch heights. High arches (like high cheekbones) were once considered a sign of elegance and sophistication. The higher arched or "cavus" foot, though has its own intrinsic problems. The high arched foot is a very poor shock absorber. If you have a high arched foot, you are more likely to suffer from knee, hip, or back pain. High arched feet can be the result of neurovascular diseases such as polio, stroke, Charcot-Marie-Tooth disease, spina bifida, and Frederich's ataxia, but are more commonly hereditary.

Metatarsal Position

Each foot contains five metatarsal bones. The area under the ends of these bones is commonly known as the "ball" of the foot. Ideally these bones should line up so that they equally distribute your body weight to the ground. In some individuals, however, the foot structure is such that one or more of the metatarsals is more plantarflexed (lower) than the others. Plantarflexed metatarsals are often referred to as "dropped" metatarsals. In some feet, the second, third, and fourth metatarsals will be lower,

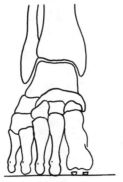

All five metatarsals hit the ground on the same level.

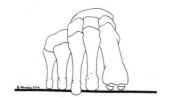

Third metatarsal is plantar flexed or "dropped."

resulting in a widespread callus on the middle part of the ball of the foot. In other cases, the first and fifth metatarsals will be "dropped" resulting in callus formation on the inside and outside portions of the ball of the foot.

One painful structural condition occurs when only one metatarsal is below the level of the others. In this instance the "dropped" metatarsal hits the ground before the other metatarsals and with greater force. This results in the formation of a localized painful corn known as an intractable plantar keratoma (IPK).

Bunions

The best known biomechanically caused foot deformity is the bunion. Technically known as hallux abducto valgus, this is another painful condition involving the big toe joint. A bunion begins as a small enlargement at the head of the first metatarsal which slowly and progressively grows.

The underlying cause of a bunion is abnormal pronation of the foot. This collapsing force gradually causes a rotational dislocation of the big toe joint. As the first metatarsal drifts toward the midline of the body, the toe itself moves in the opposite direction, often moving above or below the second toe.

Faulty foot structure leads to bunion formation. Abnormal pronation causes the foot to collapse and be unstable at a time when it should supinate and be rigid. Bunion formation is a

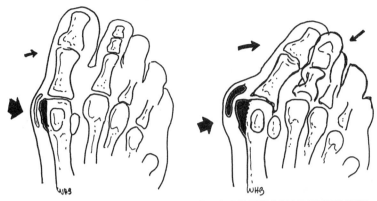

EARLY BUNION DEFORMITY   **SEVERE BUNION DEFORMITY**

gradual process which develops over many years. This condition may be hereditary and is not *caused* by wearing improper shoes. Wearing pointed shoes, will, however, *aggravate* and *accelerate* bunion formation.

Bunions cannot be *corrected* without surgery. Over the years many contraptions such as splints have been tried to correct them. People have also resorted to everything from exercise and manipulations to vitamin regimens—all in vain. The forces that cause bunions are simply too great to be mechanically corrected.

There is some evidence, however, to back up the claim that bunions can be prevented by biomechanically controlling the abnormal pronatory forces affecting the foot. These forces can

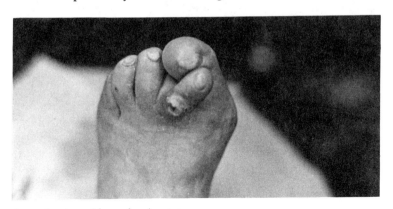

Severe bunion with overlapping toe

best be controlled by wearing orthotics, which will be discussed later in this chapter.

Diagnosis of Structural Conditions

Only in the last few decades have we begun to understand and properly diagnose biomechanical problems of the foot. As mentioned, one diagnostic tool introduced in the early eighties which holds great promise is the Electrodynagram® (EDG). The EDG is a computerized system of gait analysis.

A series of pressure sensors are attached to specific areas of a patient's foot. The patient is then asked to walk or run. Information is sent to the computer which then provides a printout including a suggested diagnosis.

A podiatrist's well-trained eye is also effective in picking up gait imperfections.

Your doctor may also take weightbearing X-rays to determine the true position of your arch as well as the functional and structural relationships of your metatarsal bones.

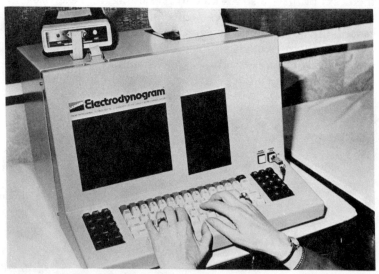

Electrodynagram® (Courtesy of Langer Biomechanics Group, Deer Park, N.Y.)

Biomechanical Management of Structural Problems

The only way to correct structural misalignments is via surgery. There are, however, biomechanical ways to *accommodate* for structural problems and thus avoid or at least delay surgery. If surgery is the only alternative, biomechanical devices can subsequently prevent a structural condition from reoccurring. The most useful of these are technically known as orthotic devices. Through common usage these have become better known as "orthotics" (although grammatically they should be called orthoses).

Orthotics

Orthotics—custom-made inserts which fit into your shoes—can be thought of as "eyeglasses" for the feet. Superficially they look like arch supports and in fact they do help support the arch, but that is only a small part of what they do. Orthotics actually change the way you walk. They prevent excess pronation of the foot and allow the foot to supinate at the proper time in the walking cycle.

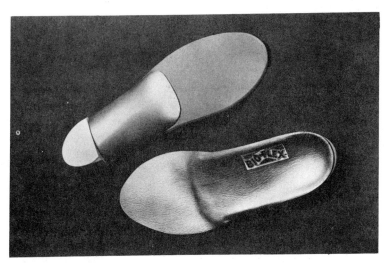

Orthotics

In the treatment of certain metatarsal conditions such as IPKs, orthotics can be modified to form depressions that will accommodate one or more "dropped" metatarsal bones. This way, a plantarflexed metatarsal which would normally hit the ground with more force than the adjacent metatarsals can now land innocently into a small depression in the orthotic. The net result is better weight distribution of the metatarsals.

Who Should Wear Orthotics

Orthotics are universally acknowledged as being useful in the treatment and prevention of many structural conditions including abnormal pronation, bunions, heels spurs, plantar fasciitis, shin splints and metatarsalgia. They are *not*, however, a panacea for all foot problems. Why?

While they provide for better foot function, orthotics do not *correct* faulty foot structure. Remember our analogy to eyeglasses—just as eyeglasses do not *correct* vision, orthotics do not correct foot structure. However, if you thought your vision wasn't up to par, you would have your vision checked. If you develop persistent foot or leg pain or notice an uneven or abnormal wear pattern on your shoes, you should visit your podiatrist or physician.

Occasionally a patient with perfectly normal feet comes into my office and asks me to make him a pair of othotics. Usually the patient has a friend who has been helped by orthotics or who has read of the benefits of wearing these devices. Wearing an orthotic unnecessarily may "over-correct" a normally functioning foot, leading to supination (outward turning of the feet, the opposite of pronation). This can actually *cause* an injury—particularly in the knees. Dr. Richard Schuster, a pioneer in the field of orthoses and director of Schuster and Richards Labs, prescribes these devices for less than forty percent of his patients.

Sports Orthotics

Orthotics have gained great popularity among athletes. During sports, the foot is subjected to many times the normal force exerted during walking. The increased forces magnify any inherent structural problem. Your foot may function normally during daily walking, but start jogging twenty-five miles a week—

the foot will hit with two to three times the amount of force exerted during walking—and suddenly you develop foot trouble. A small one-quarter inch limb length shortage (one leg is shorter than the other) becomes magnified to nearly an inch. The longer leg hits the ground harder and can result in knee, hip and back pain as the additional force is driven up the limb. A small amount of abnormal pronation which would cause little problem in walking can result in a large amount of knee pain. More than a million runners are currently wearing orthotics, and many candidly admit "without them, I'd have to give up running."

Orthotics prescribed by podiatrists are custom-made for your foot type and function. Many "over-the-counter" devices are also available, but because they are sold by shoe size, their benefits are not reliable. You may see good results if your foot type is close to that of the store model. Unfortunately, every foot is unique and people have arch height, limb length, and range of motion differences which cannot be properly addressed by a "one-size-fits-all" device. People actually send away for orthotics by mail. These so-called "custom-made" devices are made from a tracing that the patient has drawn of his foot and sent to the company. The firm then matches this drawing to the closest fitting pair of inserts available. While this method of purchasing an orthotic is slightly better than buying only by size, it still presents serious deficiencies. The foot is a three-dimensional object. It cannot be adequately represented by a two dimensional tracing. If you need orthotics and decide to invest in a pair, don't be penny wise and pound foolish.

Making An Orthotic

Before prescribing an orthotic, a podiatrist takes a careful history, noting chief complaint, shoe type, and walking habits. He or she measures the body for range of motion, angular relationships, and limb length difference, does a gait analysis, and in some cases takes weightbearing X-rays.

Casting

If the physician determines that you will benefit from orthoses, he makes a casting of your foot in its corrected position. There are many accepted ways of casting, and each orthotic laboratory suggests a particular method. However, in *all* recommended techniques, the feet are held in the proper position and plaster of Paris strips are applied to make a "negative" or model of the foot. In an old method, the foot was pressed into styrofoam contained in a cardboard box and the impression left by the foot was then filled with plaster of Paris to make a "positive" of your foot. The orthotic was then fit to this mold. The problem with this method was that the impression was made just the way the foot hit the styrofoam, without any guarantee that the foot was in the neutral position. And once it was in the foam there was no opportunity to change the foot's position.

There are two types of plaster casting techniques commonly used today. In the first method, the patient lies flat on a table and plaster strips are draped over the foot. The foot is then held in the neutral position. Proponents of this off-weightbearing position contend that this method more accurately captures the natural contour of the foot. In the second method, the patient is seated and the feet allowed to rest on a foam pad. Those using this semi-weightbearing technique believe their system more closely reflects abnormalities of the total limb.

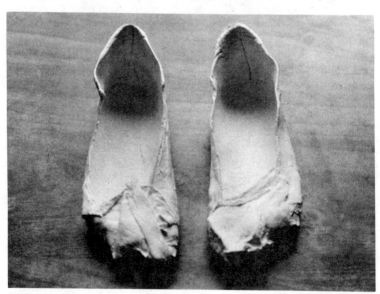

A plaster casting "negative" of the foot

Positives—models of the feet from which orthotics are made

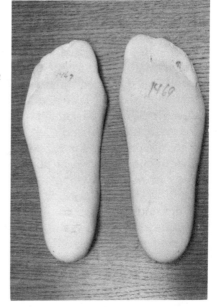

Most orthotics laboratories agree that it is essential to capture the foot with the subtalar joint (between ankle and heel bones) in a neutral position. In this position, the foot lies approximately two-thirds inverted (inward) and one-third everted (outward) and functions most efficiently. Failure to capture this position will limit the function of the orthotic, either under-correcting (pronating) or over-correcting (supinating) the foot.

The negative impression obtained from casting is sent to the laboratory where a positive is made by filling the cast shell with plaster of Paris and allowing it to dry. When the outer shell is peeled away, a plaster model of the foot remains. The orthotic device is built on the plaster form.

Materials

Choice of material can determine how well the orthotic works. Basically three types of materials are used: rigid (plastic), semi-rigid (leather), and soft (plastazote). There are advantages and disadvantages to each material.

Rigid orthotics provide the greatest pronation control, but many individuals—those with a limited range of foot motion, particularly those over thirty-five years of age, cannot wear them simply because of their rigidity.

Leather orthoses offer somewhat less control but are easier to wear because they actually mold to the foot. While they are much easier to adjust to, they do wear out more quickly and are somewhat less efficient than the plastic devices.

Plastazote orthotics provide the least control and wear out the fastest. Their chief advantages are their extreme softness (they are easy to adjust to) and their shock absorbency.

Choice of material for *your* orthotics will be dictated by your individual needs and your podiatrist's findings.

After impression casting and model making, the orthotic will be fabricated to the doctor's prescription based upon his exam findings and your chief complaint. Each orthotic lab has its own manufacturing method and its own system of quality control. Return rates for incorrectly made orthotics are low, but it is possible for a lab to make mistakes, including sending someone else's pair. Improper manufacture occurs partially because orthotics are usually handmade. Many steps involve cutting, gluing, posting and grinding. A well-made orthotic is a work of art.

The lab sends the finished product to the podiatrist, who then might make additional adjustments in your shoe, possibly removing the insole or foam arch material which, if left in, may throw a new orthotic out of balance.

Break-In Period

The podiatrist will give you a schedule for slowly breaking in the orthotics. This involves wearing them for an hour or so the first day and adding an hour or two each subsequent day until your body adjusts to them. Similarly, athletes must also "break in" orthotics slowly. A tennis player should wear orthotics for only one set during the first week and add a set each week. Runners should run a quarter of their normal distance with their orthotics on and add a comparable distance each of the next three weeks.

Breaking in orthotics too quickly can cause knee pain, back pain, or blisters. If the devices hurt, see the doctor who prescribed them. He or she may suggest that you reduce your wearing time, and then slowly increase it. Or it may be that the device needs adjustment.

Sometimes it is a combination of the wearer's impatience in not allowing proper break-in and failure to inform the doctor of discomfort so that he can make the necessary adjustments that causes the premature retirement of a basically good pair of orthotics.

Currently costing a few hundred dollars, an orthotic device represents an important, sizeable investment. The total price usually includes an exam, gait analysis, X-rays, and lab fees for producing the device itself as well as follow-up care and any necessary adjustment.

Successful use of orthotics involves several factors. To make the most out of them, orthotics should be: (1) worn only if needed; (2) made of the right material for your foot type; (3) properly cast; (4) properly manufactured; (5) adequately broken in; and (6) adjusted if necessary.

Following these fundamentals will help you get the most out of your orthotics.

The Sporting Foot   7

Athletes are the fittest group of injured people in the world. The athlete's feet have served as a testing ground for new medical treatments and products in much the same way that race cars have pioneered advances for the automotive industry.

Even the non-athlete is subject to the injuries common in athletes. Just by stepping incorrectly off a curb, you can suffer an ankle sprain similar to that suffered by a basketball player coming down from a rebound. Walk excessively on a vacation in Rome and you'll experience the same overuse syndromes of tendinitis or bursitis suffered by the marathon runner who increases training mileage too rapidly.

Sixty percent of all athletic injuries occur in the lower extremity and a majority of these affect the foot. Why? Almost all sports involve running and jumping, the trauma of which is absorbed primarily by the foot. A 150-pound athlete hits the ground with about 300–450 pounds of force. In an hour's workout, an athlete's foot is subjected to approximately five million foot-pounds of force—enough force to move a five-story building!

Most feet handle these enormous pressures admirably, but any weaknesses in *training*, *structure*, or *protection* will invariably lead to foot pain or injury.

Training Injuries

The most common training injuries result from overuse. Occurring when an individual exceeds the training capacity of his body, overuse injuries are most common in "weekend athletes"—those who suddenly gain enthusiasm for a new sport. Also affected are athletes who increase their training schedules too rapidly. A runner who has been training ten miles a week and suddenly increases his mileage to forty miles a week in anticipation of an upcoming marathon is a likely candidate as is the tennis player who has stopped playing during the winter and goes out to play three sets his first time out.

The training injury you suffer depends on which body part is the weakest or is put under the most stress. Muscles, tendons, fascia, ligaments, bones, bursa, and joints can all become injured or inflamed as a result of overuse. Many of these syndromes end with the suffix "itis," which is Latin for inflammation. Tendinitis is an inflammation of a tendon. Arthritis is an inflammation of a joint, and so forth.

Prevention

Common sense is the key in the prevention of most overuse syndromes.

1. If you're beginning a new sport or returning to an activity after a long hiatus, start out gradually.

2. Increase your level of activity gradually. Runners, for instance, should not increase mileage by more than ten percent a week.

3. Do the proper warm-up and stretches *before* working out.

4. If you are participating in an activity and experience pain, *stop and call it a day*. Pain is a device of your body's "early warning" system. If you ignore nature's warning, you may subject yourself to even further damage.

5. Set up a sensible training schedule with adequate rest days. The American College of Sports Medicine in a policy statement recommends vigorous exercise for at least one-half hour, three to five times a week. Studies have shown that working out more than five times a week does not lead to significant fitness or performance gains, but does *lead to an increase in athletic injuries.*

In general, the treatment of all overuse injuries requires Rest, Ice, Compression and Elevation—summarized by the acronym RICE.

Rest

This allows nature to heal any injured part. Depending on the severity of your injury, this can range from a decrease in activity or mileage to a complete cessation of activity. Use your best judgment.

Ice

This is the most effective way to manage most acute injuries. Ice should be applied fifteen minutes at a time to the painful or injured part, especially during the first seventy-two-hour period. Ice is preferable to heat because it also reduces swelling.

Heat and cold both cause a helpful increase in the local blood supply, but each works via a different mechanism. Heat stimulates an increase in blood flow in an attempt to cool off the skin. If, however, your circulation is diminished, heat can cause an actual burn to your skin. This is one of the reasons that heating pads are not recommended for those who have cold feet. Heat increases the "metabolic" demands on your skin. Burning of the skin can occur when your body cannot cope with this added demand.

Cold decreases the metabolic demand on your skin and causes a reflex increase in the deep blood supply. This increase is your body's attempt to warm up the skin. While frostbite is remotely possible from the use of ice, it is certainly less likely than is the possibility of a burn from the use of heat.

The best way to make a moldable icepack is to moisten a hand towel and place it into the freezer for forty-five minutes. Wrap this pack around the injured part for fifteen minutes and then return it to the freezer for another forty-five minutes. Continue this regimen until bedtime. Be sure to leave the icepack in the refrigerator overnight. If you leave it in the freezer, it will come out hard as a rock by morning.

Compression

This usually takes the form of an ace bandage or tape strapping. The objective is to reduce swelling and to restrict the range of motion of the injured part. The more severe the injury, the greater the limitation of motion required. Fractures and ligament tears, for instance, generally require cast immobilization.

Elevation

This speeds up the recovery process by allowing excess fluids to drain via gravity. One of the easiest methods of nighttime elevation is to place a few large books or telephone directories under the base of your mattress. Avoid using a pillow for elevation at night, as it invariably winds up on the floor by morning.

Beyond these basics, each of the following common athletic foot injuries presents its own particular nuances.

Achilles Tendinitis

Legend has it that the Greek warrior Achilles was invulnerable, except for a small weakness at the back of his heel. As a child, Achilles was dipped from the heels in the river Styx by his mother Thetis, making him invulnerable everywhere except at the point where she held him. Achilles met his death when Paris was able to shoot an arrow into his heel.

The Achilles tendon is aptly named, because it is the weakness of many athletes, from dancers to runners. Achilles tendinitis is an inflammation of the tendinous insertion of the calf muscles (gastrocnemius and soleus) into the back part of the heel. It is a condition characterized by pain in the posterior part of the heel which can extend upward to the calf. Individuals with shortened or tight calf muscles are particularly prone to this problem. Achilles tendinitis is commonly aggravated by any of the following factors:

1. Excessive increase in activity level, especially if running up hills, climbing, or participating in any activity in which pulling of the tendon is involved. For instance, a ballet dancer can suffer this injury as a result of coming down from *pointe*, where the relaxed tendon is pulled taut.

2. Too great a transition in heel height. Most often affected are women who go from wearing high-heeled shoes to flat sport shoes.

3. Failure to properly stretch the Achilles tendon.

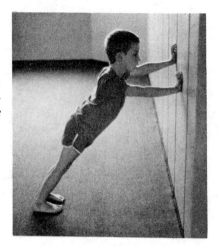

Stretching the Achilles tendon. Feet should face inwards (pigeon-toed). Do not "bounce" while stretching.

Proper stretching of the tendon is most easily done by leaning against a wall. Standing two to three feet from the wall, place both hands flat on the wall at shoulder height and lean forward at approximately a forty-five-degree angle, making sure that both heels remain flat on the ground. This stretch should be done for a minimum of three minutes before and after your activity. The tendons should be stretched slowly, by gradually increasing tension on them. Avoid bouncing, since it causes a contraction of the calf muscle.

Treatment

Treatment of Achilles tendinitis requires the basics of R.I.C.E. plus the insertion of heel lifts. A heel pad of one-half to three-quarters of an inch will relieve the pressure on the tendon and allow it to rest.

Never allow any physician to inject a steroid such as cortisone into an inflamed tendon. Once a common treatment, this is not only unnecessary but it is also outright dangerous. Studies have shown that when tendons are injected with steroids, their structure weakens, increasing the chance of future rupture.

If you are chronically plagued with Achilles tendinitis, see your sports podiatrist for further diagnosis and treatment.

Tendinitis can also occur on the top of your foot. This is generally due to either a tight-fitting shoe or a shoe on which the laces have been overtightened. This type of tendinitis usually resolves itself once a change to a properly fitting shoe is made.

Bursitis

A bursa is a balloon-like sac which cushions a tendon as it moves over a joint. When overuse occurs, these sacs fill with fluid and become painful and inflamed.

There are numerous bursae in the foot, any of which can become irritated due to overuse. The first mode of treatment after the basic R.I.C.E. is the use of a non-steroidal anti-inflammatory medication such as aspirin. Protective padding at the bursa site is also helpful, particularly when the bursa is located behind the heel. Padding provides protection from shoe irritation.

Chronic bursitis may require physical therapy and possibly the use of injectable steroids.

Arch Pain (Plantar Fasciitis)

The plantar fascia is a ligamentous band which runs under your arch from the heel to the ball of your foot. This band helps to support your arch and prevent it from collapsing under the weight of your body.

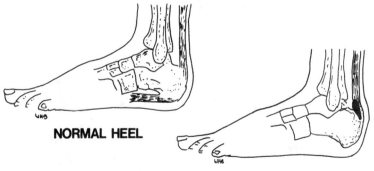

NORMAL HEEL

BURSITIS
inflammed bursal sac

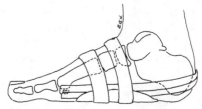

A "low dye" strapping of the foot used to support the plantar fascia

Running and jumping put an additional strain on the fascia, often causing it to become irritated, and resulting in a dull aching pain.

This condition can also affect non-athletes, particularly those who are heavy. This is due to the additional downward pressure of extra body weight which stretches the plantar ligaments.

A solidly built shoe with a rigid heel counter (see Choosing a Running Shoe) can often prevent this condition. Strapping is both a good preventive and therapeutic measure.

The most effective long-term solution to plantar fasciitis is the wearing of an orthotic, a custom-made shoe insert, which helps support your arch. Orthotics, which are made by your podiatrist, are more effective than the over-the-counter devices commonly sold in sporting goods stores (which are only sold by size). Each foot has its own "prescription" and unless you're extremely lucky, the over-the-counter device won't fit properly.

Sporthotic® (Courtesy of Langer Biomechanics Group, Deer Park, N.Y.)

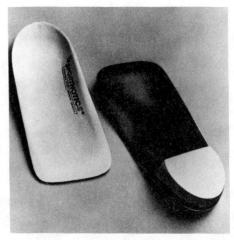

Heel Spurs

This painful condition of the heel has affected athletes from Joe DiMaggio to Billie Jean King and is somewhat related to plantar fasciitis. A spur is a piece of bone which has been gradually pulled off the bottom of the heel near the origin of the plantar fascia. This tearing occurs when the plantar fascia is over–stretched, such as when the arch is put under great stress. Heel spurs are also common in heavy non-athletes.

Heel spurs require the same prevention and treatment as plantar fasciitis: R.I.C.E., strapping, a supportive shoe, and orthotics.

When the pain in the heel is acute, injections of a steroid into the heel bursa may be indicated.

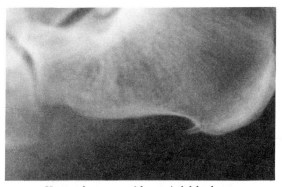

X-ray of runner with a painful heel spur

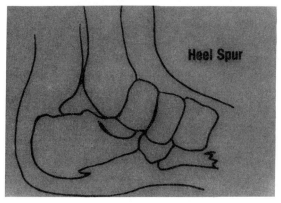

Illustration of a heel spur

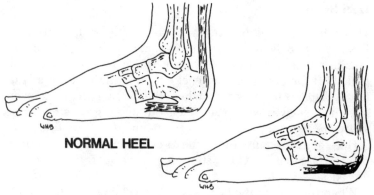

NORMAL HEEL

FASCIITIS
inflammation – heel bone muscle attachment

Foot surgery for the removal of the heel spur is a last resort, when all other conservative measures have failed. Why? The skin around the heel has a very poor blood supply. Heel spur surgery prematurely ended the brilliant career of baseball's Joe DiMaggio because his surgeon elected to perform the now-obsolete "Griffith" procedure, which involved making a large incision around DiMaggio's heel that never healed properly. Today's modern procedures involve a tiny incision and are far less traumatic.

Sever's Apophysitis

Children aged eight to fourteen often suffer heel pain due to a disruption of the growth plate at the back of the heel. This condition, known as apophysitis, is most common in children who run and jump a lot, particularly ballet dancers and gymnasts.

The back of the heel is the last part of the foot to ossify (mature). The stresses put on the heel by jumping cause the growth plate to be pulled, resulting in pain.

Taping and cushioning of the heel are two good preventive measures. Apophysitis usually subsides after the child reaches his fifteenth or sixteenth birthday. If your child is suffering from this condition, you may want to temporarily modify his athletic program until the problem is resolved. A child gymnast, for instance, might be restricted from vaulting for a few months.

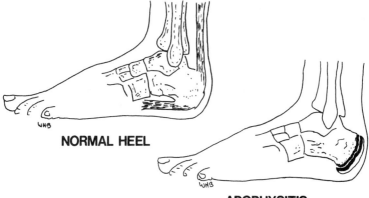

NORMAL HEEL

APOPHYSITIS
injury to bone growth plate

Fractures

A fracture of the foot or ankle is one of the most violent and dramatic sports injuries. Fractures are usually easily diagnosed. Severe pain, swelling, and discoloration (due to underlying bleeding) rapidly follow the initial trauma. Often a loud cracking sound can be heard at the time of the fracture.

Suspected fractures should be examined and X-rayed as soon as possible by a podiatrist or orthopedist. This is also true of stubbed or broken toes. A popular misconception is that broken

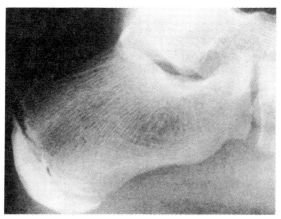

Apophysitis of the heel bone (from Radiology of the Foot, *S. Weissman)*

toes will heal themselves without treatment. This is not always the case. Hall of Fame pitcher "Dizzy" Dean was struck in the toe by a hot line drive during the 1937 all-star game. The resulting fracture forced Dean to alter his delivery and ultimately ruined his pitching arm. If a broken toe is not taped properly, it may heal crookedly, necessitating additional surgery at a future date.

Treatment of a foot fracture will require immobilization of the injured part. Major fractures require plaster casting. Minor fractures such as broken toes need only taping. Some fractures will require a combination of taping and a wooden shoe.

Stress Fractures

Less traumatic is the stress or fatigue fracture. This type of fracture falls into the category of overuse injuries and occurs when a bone is stressed past its tensile limits.

If you bend a paper clip back and forth many times, it will eventually weaken. So it is with a bone that is bent or pounded excessively (particularly on hard surfaces).

Unlike a traditional fracture, a stress fracture is difficult to diagnose. There is no severe pain and discoloration. Instead, dull aching pain, tenderness, mild swelling, and some redness are often present. The characteristic complaint of the athlete with a stress fracture is that of foot or leg pain which gets worse during activity and feels better during rest periods, only to feel worse when activity is continued.

Stress fractures are often misdiagnosed because initial X-rays are almost always negative. Only after twenty-one or more days after injury (when the body has laid down calcium in an attempt to heal the fracture) are X-rays positive.

Treatment of a stress fracture requires a combination of rest and immobilization. Stress fractures generally heal in four to eight weeks.

Shin Splints

This is a catch-all expression for many conditions which cause pain in the lower front part of the leg. Shin splints is an overuse syndrome of one or more muscles which originate on the leg and insert into the foot. The two basic conditions often found are anterior and posterior shin splints.

Anterior Shin Splints

The anterior muscles are located on the outside front part of the leg. They act to slow down and prevent the foot from slapping the ground. These muscles can become irritated when an athlete begins to train on hills or changes from a flatfooted to a toe-running style.

Anterior shin splints are often predisposed by a relative weakness of the front leg muscles. Activities such as running tend to build up the calf muscles more than the anterior leg muscles. Studies have shown that when the calf muscles become more than four-and-a-half times stronger than the anterior leg muscles, the development of shin splints is likely.

Prevention of anterior shin splints is accomplished by exercising these muscles. If you religiously exercise them, you will gradually build them up and avoid the muscle fatigue and inflammation of anterior shin splints.

The exercise that is most effective in building up these muscles is dorsi-flexion of the foot. In a sitting position, stretch the front part of your foot up toward your leg, as if trying to touch your shin with your toes. This exercise should be done in three sets of ten repetitions each day. After the first week, you may begin to add a one pound weight per week for the next five weeks. You needn't use standard weights. A few books in a pail can be hung over your foot.

Treatment of anterior shin splints consists of R.I.C.E. plus the avoidance of hill-running or hard surfaces.

Posterior Shin Splints

This type of shin splint is an irritation of the posterior tibial muscle at its origin in the lower inside part of the leg. This is a deep muscle which inserts into the arch area and helps support the foot. When the foot excessively pronates (the arch flattens), this muscle is stressed, causing fatigue and pain.

Supportive shoes, strapping, and/or orthotic shoe inserts generally resolve this type of shin splint.

Ankle Sprains

This condition borders on being both a training and a structural injury. Ankle sprains are certainly among the most commonly suffered injuries of athletes. They are more common in individuals with a large range of ankle motion. If you can easily invert your feet (turn the soles toward each other) your chances of a sprain are increased.

Sprains are not easy to prevent. Most occur when your foot plants in an incorrect position. If you have a tendency to sprain your ankles often, stable low heeled shoes, strapping, and elastic ankle supports can be helpful.

The treatment for an ankle sprain depends on the severity of the injury. A minor ligament pull requires little treatment. If after a few minutes, you can hop on the injured foot without pain, it's safe for you to return to your activity.

If you *can't* bear weight without pain you will need R.I.C.E. and a further work-up. In a moderate ankle sprain, a tear often occurs in the lateral talo-fibular ligament. Tears of this nature should not be taken lightly. Because of the poor blood supply to this area, ligament injuries may take even longer to heal than bone fractures.

In severe ankle sprains the calcaneal-fibular ligament may also be severed. Treatment of this type of sprain ranges from casting to surgery (to resew the torn ligaments).

STRUCTURAL INJURIES:

Limb Length Difference

Foot, knee, leg, hip, and back pain felt on *one side* of the body can often be the result of a difference in the length of the limb and studies have shown that approximately nine out of ten individuals have a measurable limb length difference. A shortened limb can be hereditary or may stem from back problems such as scoliosis (a curvature of the spine).

There are some simple ways of detecting limb length difference. When you have your clothes hemmed do you have to take up one side more than the other? Look in the mirror. Is one shoulder higher than the other? Inspect the bottom of a well worn sneaker. Is one side more worn than the other? Chances are the longer limb is hitting harder and wearing out the sole faster.

In most cases, because the longer limb hits harder and therefore transmits more force to that side, pain due to a limb length difference will be present in that longer limb.

A limb length difference can also result if one foot pronates (collapses) more than the other. This collapsing tends to shorten the foot and limb.

Limb length problems are more severe in the athlete than the non-athlete. A quarter inch difference may not cause any symptoms in the non-athlete, but the athlete with that same quarter inch difference will experience pain because he is contacting the ground with two to three times the force of the non-athlete. His quarter inch shortage becomes in effect a one-half to three-quarter inch shortage. Runners have been known to actually limp without even knowing it. Have a friend observe you as you run. Are your arms swinging symmetrically or is one arm swinging faster to compensate for balance?

Structural limb length differences are easily managed through the use of either a heel lift or an orthotic insert.

Functional Limb Length Difference

Functional limb length differences result from running on uneven surfaces such as an indoor banked track. In this situation, the inner foot is subjected to greater force than the outer foot. Running on the beach exerts this type of pressure (the average beach slopes about fourteen degrees) as can running on the street, since most roads are banked for drainage.

The logical solution to functional limb problems is to alternate directions when running, thus equalizing the force on both limbs.

Knee Pain

Knee pain associated with athletic participation is often caused by structural foot problems. Many times an athlete comes into my office complaining of both foot and knee pain, very often not making the connection between these problems.

The knee is basically a hinge joint designed to move only in an up and down direction (flexion/extension). The smooth operation of the knee assumes that the foot will be stable to the ground. If the foot pronates (collapses) the leg rotates inward, causing the knee to move from side to side (obliquely). This abnormal motion causes the cartilage under the kneecap to wear unevenly, resulting in the common and painful knee injury, chondromalacia patellae, often referred to as "runner's knee."

Chondromalacia patellae responds well to orthotic inserts which prevent the foot from excessively pronating.

PROTECTION BASED INJURIES:

Blisters

Almost everyone has experienced the painful and annoying lesions resulting from excessive friction and pressure on skin commonly known as blisters. While they may be considered a minor affliction by some, you can be sure that Jimmy Connors doesn't agree. During the 1979 Grand Prix Master's tennis tournament, a painful foot blister forced him to default and cost him an almost certain $100,000 first prize. You may never find yourself in Connors' position, but taking proper care of your blisters will prevent the pain and disability of an infected blister.

Prevention

To prevent blisters, you have to eliminate friction. One of the prime sources of friction is a shoe which fits improperly. If you find that your shoes are causing friction, you can modify them by making slits above the area of the blister formation.

Spenco Second Skin® is an over-the-counter product which can be applied to the areas on your foot which chronically form blisters.

If your skin is either too dry or too sweaty, you will also have a tendency to form blisters. If your skin is dry, apply a thin coat of petroleum jelly to your foot before activity. If your foot tends to sweat, a little cornstarch added to your shoe and/or sock may be helpful.

Treatment

Small blisters require the least care. Apply ice to them for a few minutes, then cover them with a bandage. *Never remove the blis-*

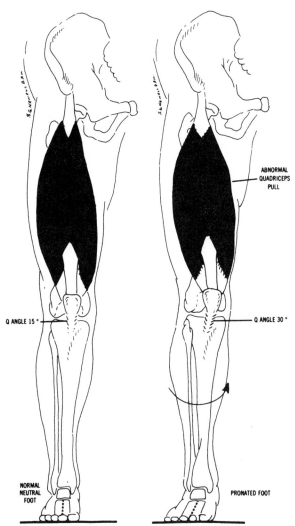

Pronation and knee pain (from Podiatric Sports Medicine)

ter's overlying skin. This acts as a barrier against bacteria and aids in the prompt healing of the blister.

For large and painful blisters, more care is required:

1. Sterilize a new sewing needle, either by cleaning it with 70% isopropyl alcohol, heating it with a match, or by placing it in a pressure cooker for a few minutes.

2. Clean the area around the blister with an antiseptic such as alcohol or Betadine®.

3. Make many small punctures in the blister to allow fluid to escape. Blot this fluid with a small piece of sterile gauze.

4. Apply a topical antibiotic ointment such as Mycitracin® or Bacitracin® to the blister site.

5. Cover the blister with a protective pad.

6. If the blister contains blood or becomes infected, see your doctor.

Black and Blue Toenails

This condition, technically known as subungual hematoma is a painful and unattractive condition of the nails which is caused by the accumulation of blood under the nails and occurs when the nails bang against the shoe during activity.

Prevention

Prevention of this condition requires the selection of a shoe with adequate length and toe box height. If this condition happens to you often, try buying the next size shoe or a style with a higher toe box.

Existing shoes can be salvaged by making a slit in the upper at the point where the nail contacts. With your shoes on, make a mark at the point where you feel the offending nail. Now remove the shoe and make a vertical slit where you made your mark.

Keeping your nails as short as possible is another effective method of preventing black toenails.

Treatment

Painful hematomas should be drained. You can do this yourself in much the same way you would drain a blister, that is, by using a sterile pin to make several holes in the nail, but a podiatrist or physician can usually perform the procedure less painfully and more effectively.

How to Choose an Athletic Shoe

Confused about buying a good pair of athletic shoes? No wonder! Sales of athletic shoes have soared in the last decade and there are currently hundreds of different styles and shapes available. This is not only attributable to the increased number of people engaged in physical activity, but also to the new social acceptability of these shoes for casual wear. From blue suede leather to dayglow orange nylon mesh, athletic shoes have become a staple of every fashionable wardrobe.

The evolutionary root of today's training shoe was a croquet shoe used by the upper class around the turn of the twentieth century. This shoe has subsequently undergone modification to produce cleated soccer, football, baseball, and golf shoes, spiked sprinting shoes, high topped basketball, boxing, and wrestling shoes as well as the ever-popular tennis sneaker. The term sneaker became popular because its quiet rubber sole made it possible to "sneak up" on someone without being heard.

Most sports medicine authorities agree that the basic training shoe is the most versatile general sports shoe. Following the 1960 Olympic games, German athletic companies began advertising these shoes for sale to the general public. The Olympic Committee frowned on the practice of portraying athletes wearing name brand shoes and there was quite an uproar about athletes accepting compensation for this type of endorsement. The idea, however, was successful. Thus started the fierce competition among manufacturers to capture an increasing share of a rapidly growing market. Athletic shoes became the "chic" thing to wear during the 1979 New York City Transit strike. Now it seems that everybody (from supermarkets to high-class boutiques) is selling training shoes.

Unfortunately, many of these shoes have numerous shortcomings. No shoe can be expected to fit all feet or perform best for all sports. If you specialize in an individual sport, you should purchase a shoe designed for that sport. The characteristics of a specific sport shoe will be determined by the motions used in that sport.

Activities such as running and jogging most often involve unidirectional motion (straight ahead). Tennis, raquetball, and ping-pong require a great deal of lateral motion. Basketball, soccer, and football involve both unidirectional and lateral motion.

The more linear your sport, the stiffer the sides of your shoes should be. The more lateral the sport, the more twist should be possible in the shoe. A simple way to test this characteristic is to hold the shoe in your hand and twist it as if you were wringing out a towel. A tennis shoe should twist easily; a running shoe should not.

Fitting Variables

Each shoe company uses its own lasts (models of the foot) over which they construct their shoes. One company's shoe may fit you comfortably, while another company's same size shoe will not. There may be no shoe which fits your foot perfectly. Only comparative fittings of different styles and sizes will assure you of the best possible fit. Some companies such as New Balance produce athletic shoes both in wide and narrow widths. The shoe last type will also be a factor.

Last Type

Two types of construction are commonly used in the manufacture of an athletic shoe; board lasting and slip lasting. You can determine the method used by examining the inside bottom of the shoe.

Board lasted shoes have a cardboard insert glued into the bottom of the shoe which adds greater rigidity to the shoe. Slip lasted shoes have no board, making the shoe somewhat lighter and less supportive. If you examine a slip lasted shoe carefully, you will notice the stitch marks where the bottom has been sewn together. Slip lasted shoes are generally lighter and less expensive for the shoe manufacturer to produce.

The choice of which last type you should choose depends on the amount of support and shoe stability you need and the amount of weight you are willing to tolerate. Board lasted shoes are best for support and stability, but somewhat heavier than slip lasted shoes.

Last Shape

Two basic last shapes are available; straight and curved (inflare).

The last shape is an important factor in determining whether your shoe will fit properly, yet few people ever bother to check whether a particular shoe or sneaker matches the shape of their foot. Many people buy shoes by brand name or on the recommendation of a friend or athletic magazine. I'm often asked, "What is the best shoe?" Unfortunately, there is no one best shoe for everyone. A particular Nike might be best for your foot, while a particular Adidas or Saucony might be best for your friend.

You can compare your foot shape to the sole by placing the bottom of the shoe against the bottom of your foot. Does your foot match the shape closely? An efficient method for doing this is to make a tracing of your foot before visiting the local sporting shoe store. Cut out the tracing and bring this model of your foot to the store. Now you can rapidly compare this tracing to any of the dozens of available shoes on display to find out which brands and models match most closely. With the high cost of athletic shoes, it pays to select wisely.

Quality Control

Most sport shoes are mass produced, often in Korea, Taiwan, and Hong Kong. Quality control can often be a problem. Examine each pair of shoes carefully before you buy them. Look for obvious defects such as loose stitching, or improperly glued parts. Next place the shoes on a flat surface. If you can rock the shoe from side to side, find another pair. Look at the counter of the shoe. It should be perfectly level.

Heel Height

The heel height of an athletic shoe is another variable in your fitting. Athletes with short calf muscles or a history of Achilles tendinitis should look for the highest heel available. Many athletic shoe manufacturers are now incorporating a heel lift into their shoes. If you can't easily touch your toes from a standing position, you should benefit from increased heel height.

Heel Counter

The heel counter is found in the back part of the shoe. It functions to provide support for the heel bone on ground contact. The counter should be as rigid as possible. You can test the counter strength by holding the shoe flat in your hand and attempting to bend the counter forward with three fingers. If the counter bends easily, look for a better shoe.

Shock Absorption

A good training shoe should provide as much protection to your foot as possible. The shock absorption layer is usually found directly above the bottom or wear layer. Some companies use different colors to distinguish each sole layer. The shock absorption layer should provide good cushioning, without completely collapsing. It may be difficult to determine how good a shoe absorbs shock without running in it. Some athletic magazines run such tests on shoes, and it may be a good idea to contact them if you aren't certain about the particular shock absorption of a specific model.

Sole Flexibility

The front part of the sole (where the foot bends) should be flexible. Take the shoe in one hand and with the other hand attempt to flex the sole upward. Keep in mind that your legs must undergo the same effort and motion during running. Too stiff a sole means wasted effort. If you can't flex the sole easily, the sole is not flexible enough.

Toe Box

Look for a shoe with a high toe box. Adequate space in the front part of the shoe provides room for the toes to flex during the propulsive phase of running. If the toe box is too low, the toes

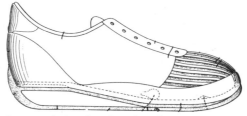

This athletic shoe was designed with a pleated upper to prevent the common problem of black and blue toenails (Block & Beekman, 1982)

bang and scrape against the top of the shoe, leading to blisters, broken toenails, and black and blue toes. This is particularly important if you wear a sports orthotic.

Recently, a shoe was designed with a novel approach to toe box height. A pleated upper was used to allow for the expansion of the toe during sports activity.

Inner Cushioning

The shoe must also have ample inner cushioning. This provides for proper shock absorption within the shoe. Put your hand into your shoe and press down on the sole. There should be some give. Many athletic shoe manufacturers add Spenco type inner soles for this purpose.

Arch Supports

Many athletes are concerned with arch support, but what most shoe companies advertise as arch supports (small foam pads) are not functional. How much support can sponge rubber provide to a 150-pound athlete? Recently some shoe companies have included "orthotic-type" foam inserts in their running shoes. While these are better than foam arch supports, they still are a long way from being functional orthotics. There is simply no way to mass produce an arch support that will fit everyone's arch. If you require arch support you should see a sports oriented podiatrist who will probably rip out the prefabricated arch from your shoe and replace it with something more substantial.

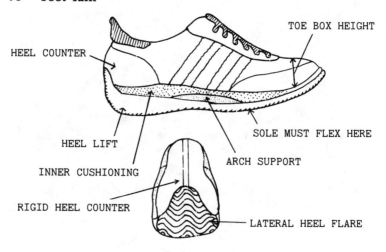

HEEL COUNTER

TOE BOX HEIGHT

SOLE MUST FLEX HERE

HEEL LIFT

INNER CUSHIONING

ARCH SUPPORT

RIGID HEEL COUNTER

LATERAL HEEL FLARE

Cost

You don't always get what you pay for. Athletic shoes currently are priced from about fifteen to well over one hundred dollars, and the most expensive shoe is not always the best one for you. On the other hand, don't be baited by sales, particularly of unknown brands. Consider your shoes important equipment. Find the shoe with the best features and which feels most comfortable.

Replacing Worn Sports Shoes

After a while, your once new athletic shoes will begin to look old and you'll want to replace them. The question is "when?" Because many athletic shoes cost over a hundred dollars a pair, you'll want to make them last as long as possible.

The first parameter to look at is sole wear. A worn sole is not by itself reason enough to replace a shoe. Most athletic shoe stores as well as shoe repair outlets are equipped to resole your shoes, generally at a small fraction of the cost of a new pair. If you check the classified sections of any running or tennis magazine, you will also find similar services.

The sole layers of many sports shoes are color coded to indicate which is the wear layer (usually the black layer on the bottom) and the shock absorption layer (usually the lighter colored layer above the wear layer). When you notice that the colored layer is beginning to show through, it's time to replace or rebuild the sole. Rebuilding can be accomplished by applying a product such as Shoe-Goo® to the sole.

If the heel counter is shot, be prepared to buy a new shoe soon. You may be able to extend the useable life of the shoe somewhat by adding a plastic M-F Heel cup or a Tuli® Heel cup (both available in most sporting goods stores). A breakdown in the heel counter indicates a decrease in the total structural integrity of the shoe.

If the upper part of the shoe begins to separate from the sole, there's not much you can do. Start shopping!

If you are happy with your old pair of shoes, it makes sense to replace them with the same model. This is sometimes difficult because athletic shoe companies tend to believe that "new is always better." European manufacturers are sometimes wiser. Karhu, a Finnish company has produced the same model (#2323) for at least 10 years. It was a superior shoe when it was first introduced, and it remains so today, despite the numerous "improvements" of other shoe manufacturers.

The Young Foot 8

From their birth, we are concerned about our children's feet. We breathe a sigh of relief when we see their "ten fingers and ten toes." We marvel at the newborn's exquisitely tiny feet . . . how flexible they are, how agile.

A baby can grasp with his feet. The feet and hands have not yet greatly differentiated in the newborn, so a baby will try to suck his toes as well as his fingers. He will often extend a foot instead of a hand to grasp an object.

Walking

The process of learning to walk is truly miraculous. You may remember the riddle of the sphinx: "What starts off with four legs, then has only two legs and finally three legs?" The answer, of course, is man—we start on all fours, progress to bipedal walking and eventually require a cane (the third leg) to get around. Most parents are concerned about how soon and how well their child will walk, and some well-meaning parents may attempt to speed up "Mother Nature" by putting shoes on a non-walking child. Actually this only hampers and delays the normal walking process. A baby should be allowed to wiggle his toes and explore the world with his feet. This is how he gains an early sense of position. Remember that until relatively recent times, shoes for babies were unheard of. So, do not try to rush your child into early walking. Ignore your next-door-neighbor's triumphant description of her Johnny's first steps. A child normally begins to walk unassisted when he is ready. This will occur between the ages of eight and eighteen months. There is no safe way that a parent can substantially speed up the internal "walking clock" of a child and you can do damage if you try to. Why?

Initially a baby's foot structure is not mature enough to support the child's weight. Most of the future foot bones are still cartilagenous. The ligaments of the foot are still loose due to the presence of the hormone relaxin in the baby's bloodstream—a hormone originally produced by the pregnant mother to relax the ligaments of the pelvis during labor. Pressure on these highly malleable structures can flatten out the foot and create a problem for life.

Flatfeet or "Fat" Feet

All babies' feet appear flat. Most, however, are merely fat. Nature has provided the infant's foot with an ample fat pad which serves to cushion and protect the baby during creeping and crawling. If you have a question as to whether your infant has flat feet, have him examined by a podiatrist, pediatrician, or orthopedist. If the infant is found to have congenital flatfoot, treatment should be started as soon as possible.

Years ago, flatfeet in children was treated with arch support devices known as "cookies." These devices have been replaced by orthotics, which are custom-made shoe inserts. Orthotics are far superior to "cookies" because they support the entire foot, not just the arch. For more information on orthotics see page 69.

Those Dangerous Infant Walkers

The wide use of infant walkers poses a substantial danger to a baby's welfare. A child standing in a walker before he is standing on his own is putting entirely too much stress on his foot structures. In addition, walkers have caused children serious injuries from falls down flights of stairs. Walkers give parents the false impression that their children are safely occupied, but without appropriate supervision, children in walkers have reached counters with medicines, knives and other dangerous objects.

In addition, Dr. Richard L. Saphir, a prominent pediatrician at

Manhattan's Mt. Sinai Hospital points out that "there appears to be no evidence that children who used walkers ultimately walked earlier than children who didn't. Overuse of walkers on the other hand prevents a child from adequately experiencing the crawling stage so necessary for healthy development, good-body image and coordination."

Foot problems begin in utero. Some are hereditary. If the parent suffers from a particular problem or has an awkward walk, the child should be screened early for foot problems. Often the position of the baby in the uterus causes cramping of the foot structures and interferes with normal growth and development. A seemingly minor imperfection at birth, often not apparent to the parent, can progress with time.

We mentioned that the flexibility and agility of the baby's feet, combined with an overanxious parent's attempts to have the child walking early can cause structural damage. Flexibility and agility however, are advantageous to the child who already has a foot disorder. Defects when picked up shortly after birth can often be treated by simple manipulation and specified exercises. The longer these deformities go untreated, the more extensive and traumatic the correction will be. By several months of age an orthopedic device is normally needed to correct rotations of the hip, leg and foot.

With the passage of time, these treatments become less and less useful and the child's feet may have to be set in a cast. If left untreated for longer periods, surgery or the lifelong use of orthotics might be the only way to insure proper gait.

It is wise for a parent who is concerned about his child's foot development to seek out the advice of a podiatrist or orthopedist. Pediatricians are often not as concerned as they should be about a child's feet, partly because they are treating the entire child and partly because they are very sensitive about alarming the parents. Also, the pediatrician will most likely not be seeing that child when any foot problems become more evident in his teen and adult years.

Very often, too, the child develops in ways which accommodate for the problem. Sports in which the child does not function well are avoided. Often he or she is not even aware of foot limitations. Quite often the child outgrows the pediatrician but not the problem.

Some hospitals recognize the need for early detection of foot problems and have podiatrists on staff who routinely examine the newborn.

Examination of the Newborn

Shortly after birth the child should be examined by an orthopedist or podiatrist. Structural problems such as a congenitally dislocated hip or clubfoot can be treated much more easily if they are diagnosed early. As a parent, *you* can also examine your infant periodically. When you change the baby's diaper, look at him closely. Are both sides of the body symmetrical? Are both legs and feet mirror images of each other? Now turn your tot on his stomach. Look again for symmetry. Are there the same number of skin folds on each thigh? The answer to all these questions should be *yes*. If you notice anything unusual, have it checked out by your pediatrician. If treatment is indicated, he will likely send you to an orthopedist or podiatrist specializing in young children.

Some Normal Findings

It may be comforting for you to know that children undergo some normal structural changes about which you need not be concerned. The knee position of children, for example, will change over time. At birth, all normal children will be bowlegged. This condition will gradually reduce so that by age two the position of the child's knee will be straight. From two through six the position of the knees will normally become knock-kneed. From ages six to twelve the tendency will again shift to straight knees.

Look to your parents for guidance in these matters. Did you or your spouse have a particular structural condition like in-toe or out-toe? Did you "outgrow" the problem or do you still have the same condition? The answers are important. If you outgrew a structural problem, chances are that your child will do the same. If your foot problem continued into adulthood (and most foot conditions are hereditary) treatment for you child's problem is indicated.

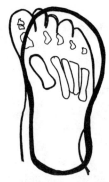

Metatarsus adductus. *The foot is superimposed over a normal shoe.*

Metatarsus Adductus

This is a structural condition of the foot in which the metatarsal bones bend inward giving the foot a "comma" shape. If it is diagnosed early enough, painless, non-invasive methods of treatment can be instituted. These include stretching exercises and corrective shoes. By the age of four months, serial casting may be necessary. In this procedure, the doctor uses plaster of paris splints to hold the baby's feet in the proper position. These casts are changed every few weeks until the position of the foot is straight. If metatarsus adductus is not treated early enough, surgery may eventually be necessary. So, once again, early detection of any foot abnormality is crucial.

In-Toe Gait

In-toe or pigeon toe gait is a condition in which the child's feet turn inward. This causes the child to fall frequently. There is a tendency for in-toe to reduce somewhat as one gets older, so it's a good idea to check whether you or your spouse had the condition and whether the condition was outgrown.

It is necessary to find out at what level the toeing-in is being caused. Internal rotation of the hips, internal torsion of the legs, or metatarsus adductus are all potential causes. You can determine exactly where the problem is by checking the position of your child's knees as he walks. If the knees point straight, the

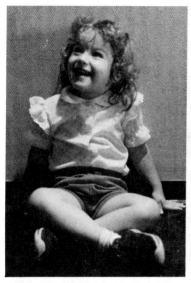 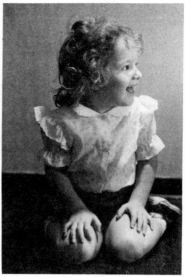

The proper way to sit "Indian Style"   Don't allow your child to sit this way

problem is below the knees. If the knees point in, the problem is in the hip.

Sitting position plays a significant role in the management of in-toe. Children who "sit on their haunches with their legs un-der them tend to worsen the condition. Conversely, sitting "In-

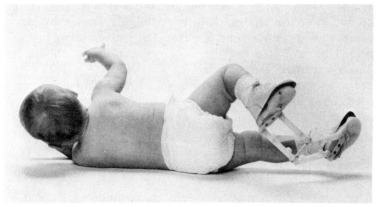

Counter rotational splint (courtesy of Langer Group, Deer Park, N.Y.)

dian" style with crossed legs is one of the best exercises to stretch the hip muscles and correct the condition.

One of the most popular orthopedic treatments of this condition has been the use of the Denis-Browne bar. This is a splint worn at night which externally rotates the legs and hips. However, bars are not effective in treating foot conditions such as metatarsus adductus. In fact, the bar may actually damage the feet by flattening the arches. A newly introduced device which holds great promise is the Counter-Rotational Splint®. This device, designed by Dr. Paul Jordon, allows the foot to be manipulated independently of the upper limb.

Out-Toe

Some children walk with an out-toe position. This is often a result of abnormal pronation, the collapsing of the arch of the foot. Children under one year of age with this condition will often benefit from serial casting. Children older than one year will benefit from the wearing of orthotics, which serve to support the arch while holding the foot in the proper position.

Out-toe may also be caused by external rotation of the hips. In these cases the use of exercises and Denis-Browne bars may be useful.

Bowlegs

This is a condition in which the distance between the knees is greater than the ankles. This is technically known as genu varum and is normal until age two. Bowlegs are often accompanied by an in-toe gait. In these cases treatment should be directed at the in-toe condition.

Bow legs seldom require drastic measures. Splints have been used, but with only limited success.

Knock Knees

Knock Knees are a normal condition from approximately age two to six.

After age six this condition should gradually decrease. Flatfeet due to abnormal pronation are often associated with knock

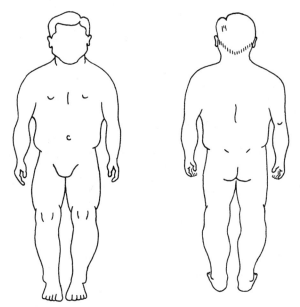

Bowlegs. Note that the feet are closer together than the knees.

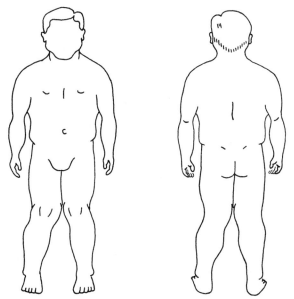

Knock knees. Note that the knees are closer together than the feet.

knees. In this situation, the abnormal pronation should be treated with orthotic devices.

Toe Walking

There are several reasons that a child might walk on his toes. Tight calf muscles are a common cause and proper stretching of the calf muscles will usually correct the gait. If the child does not "come down" after a few weeks of stretching, he should receive a complete neurological examination. Neurological diseases such as cerebral palsy can result in a toe walking gait.

Selecting Children's Shoes

Your children deserve to wear the best shoes that you can find for them. Their feet are rapidly growing and at a stage when wearing improper shoes can exert a deforming force on them. Unfortunately the many misconceptions about the buying of children's shoes often make it difficult to know which shoes are best for your child.

Your Child's First Shoes

As mentioned earlier, there is no reason to buy shoes for your child before he can walk. Soft booties are acceptable for protection from the cold but *not* for walking. Your toddler's first pair of footwear does not have to be shoes! Sneakers will do fine providing they meet the same criteria of good shoes. The most important of these standards is that *the sole be extremely flexible*. This flexibility is necessary to insure proper walking. You should be able to flex the front sole of the shoe with just two fingers' pressure. Remember your child may only weigh twenty pounds. If the sole of the shoe is thick, it may actually take more force than the child's weight to bend it!

The next consideration should be the strength of the counter. This is the part of the shoe which surrounds the heel. The counter provides much of the support of the shoe and should be as stiff as possible. If you can easily bend the counter down (like in the "old style" sneaker) look for another pair.

A popular misconception is that young children require "high top" shoes. The reason usually given was that these shoes gave the child added ankle support. But the truth is that the child will develop the muscles and ligaments which provide ankle stability without "high top" shoes. These shoes, while providing good ankle support, might actually *delay* the child's development of stable ankles.

Finding the Proper Size

Children's feet grow rapidly. It must be the parent's decision as to when shoes need to be replaced. This can be a bit unpredictable because children's feet tend to grow in spurts. It is possible to have your child fitted for a specific size shoe and have him outgrow it in two or three weeks. This can be quite distressing since the cost of quality children's shoes is nearly as much as that of adult shoes.

Some parents try to save money by "passing down" shoes from older children or relatives. This is a poor idea. Every child "wears in" a shoe differently, and while the size of the shoe may be the same, the molding effect on the shoe from the way each child walks varies. Another factor to consider is that the structural strength of a used shoe is likely to be poor.

One acceptable way of increasing the wearable life of a shoe is to buy a slightly larger size. It is certainly better to err in this direction than to choose a smaller shoe. If you go this route, aim to buy a shoe a half-size larger than the actual measured size of the foot. Also check that the child's foot is not coming out of the shoe and the child does not trip while walking.

AGE	CHECK SHOE SIZE
2–6	every 1 to 2 months
6–10	every 2 to 3 months
10–12	every 3 to 4 months
12–15	every 4 to 5 months
15–20	every 6 months
over 20	every time shoes are purchased.

The Footwear Council offers these fitting tips between shoe purchases:

1. If the child takes off his shoes repeatedly, this may indicate that the shoes are too small.

2. Any sign of a limp could mean trouble, and shoes should be checked.

3. If the lining of the shoe shows excessive wear in the area of the fifth toe, the shoes are too short. Feel inside for dents from toe pressure on the lining.

4. Watch for red marks across the top of the toes and on the sides of the child's foot. That indicates pressure from the shoe.

5. Check to see if soles are unevenly worn, showing excessive wear on the inner or outer edges. Also check heels of the shoes for uneven wear. These could be indications of foot or ankle problems and in this case, the child should be taken to an expert fitter for corrective shoes.

6. Don't pass shoes along to other children—children's feet are malleable and you can pass along fitting problems with the shoes. Leather shoes conform to the shape of the feet of the wearer which will prevent them fitting the feet of a second wearer.

Growing Pains

The process of growing is not painful. What has become known as "growing" pain is usually simple muscle fatigue. The amount of exercise a healthy child does is staggering. Try duplicating your child's activity and you'll likely experience some "growing" pains of your own.

Muscle fatigue should be treated symptomatically. Warm baths and massages work well. Tylenol® or similar medications may also be useful. If pain continues, see your pediatrician or podiatrist. Muscle fatigue may also be related to poor foot structure. If your child is flatfooted, for instance, his leg muscles will fatigue while overworking in an attempt to hold up his arch. Orthotics are useful in eliminating this type of muscle fatigue.

Limping

There are many reasons that your child might begin to limp. Injury is the most common, so you should carefully examine your child for evidence of trauma. Stepping on a foreign body such as a piece of glass or wood splinter are also common reasons for limping. Plantar warts should also be looked for. These virus-induced growths are most often found on the bottom of the foot and generally appear in the fall months. To learn more about warts see page 41.

Sometimes a child limps for unknown reasons. This clinical entity first dubbed the "ten day limp" by Dr. Herman Tax suddenly appears and disappears without known cause. If your child begins to limp and you can't find a reason, you would do well to remember this syndrome before panicking.

The Foot as a Mirror of General Health   9

Did your physician ever ask you to "take everything off except your socks"? If he did, he might have missed an opportunity to gain some valuable diagnostic information. Your feet have a lot to say about how healthy the rest of the body is.

Are your ankles ever swollen? This could be a sign of congestive heart failure. Are your feet insensitive to pain or temperature? These are signs found in diabetes as well as other conditions which affect the neurovascular system. Do your feet always feel cold? This is a common symptom of circulatory disease. Are your nails clubbed? This can be a sign of chronic respiratory disease.

As you can see, the feet hold tremendous diagnostic significance for conditions elsewhere in the body. This is partially due to their anatomical position. The feet are gravitationally the lowest part of the body and therefore any excess fluids accumulated in the body will ultimately end up there. This explains why congestive heart failure results in swollen ankles and feet. In this condition the heart is not strong enough to pump all the fluid returning to it from the veins. Swollen feet are an early sign which can be easily missed. Later on in the disease, fluid accumulates in the lungs making breathing difficult.

The vessels providing circulation to the feet are among the smallest in the body. Diseases such as arteriosclerosis (hardening of the arteries) also affect the feet early. Cold feet are an early sign of such diseases.

Generally speaking, any disease resulting in the loss of pain sensation will likely be manifested early on in the foot, thereby creating a condition known as a "neurotrophic" foot. Among these are arteriosclerosis, diabetes, Charcot-Marie-Tooth disease, syphilis, and stroke. What would it feel like to suffer from a neurotrophic foot? If a healthy foot's shoes fit improperly, a blister could develop that would prompt you to remove the offending shoe. The individual with a neurotrophic foot, however, would not even feel the blister. He would continue to wear the shoe, possibly causing extensive trauma to the foot. By the time he realized the extent of the problem, a deep infection may have set in. Such feet easily develop open sores known as ulcers, which heal with great difficulty.

Diabetes

A systemic disease with a special predilection for the feet is diabetes mellitus, a metabolic disorder in which the body is not able to transport sugar from the blood to the tissues.

Diabetes causes a thickening of the small vessels in the body, some of which supply the nerve fibers. When these vessels close, the underlying area becomes insensitive to pain and temperature.

The foot is of particular concern to diabetics because it is so vulnerable to trauma and its vessels are so small. Diabetics are very prone to both foot infections and ulcers and should therefore be seen regularly by both a physician and a podiatrist.

Diabetes tends to run in families. If a member of your family has diabetes, you should periodically have your blood tested. Also be aware of some of the general symptoms of this disease: increased thirst, frequent urination, fatigue, recent loss in weight, generalized itching, weakness, and dryness of the skin.

If you are a diabetic or suffer from any disease which results in decreased pain and temperature sensation, you should:

1. Monitor water temperature. Be sure to use a thermometer to measure the temperature of water when bathing. If you step into a hot tub, you may unknowingly burn your feet. The recommended temperature for bathing is ninety to ninety-five degrees Fahrenheit.

2. Inspect your feet daily. Look for signs of redness and swell-

ing. These are signs of inflammation or infection. Cuts, abrasions, or cracks in the skin must be treated promptly with an antiseptic solution such as Betadine® and covered with dry sterile gauze. Use only paper tape to secure gauze. *Never* use conventional adhesive tape. Removal of such tape can be dangerous because of the possibility of also removing the top layer of skin.

3. Keep the skin of your feet—and your entire body—moist and supple. Regular application of a moisturizing skin cream helps prevent your skin from drying out and cracking.

4. Buy the softest and best fitting shoes possible. Properly fitting shoes are essential in the prevention of pressure sores and ulcers. Any new pair of shoes must be "broken in" slowly. Wear a new pair a half hour the first day and add an additional half hour each subsequent day. Inspect your feet after each wearing. Look for signs of redness or irritation. If such friction marks are found, immediately note their presence and bring the shoes to your shoe repairer for modification. Custom molded shoes are recommended for those who have difficulty in finding shoes to properly fit their feet.

5. Never attempt to cut your toenails. The circulation to the toes is among the poorest in the body. If you cut yourself, an infection may ensue. Many limbs have had to be amputated as a result of gangrene which resulted from such infections. Podiatrists are specially trained to cut the nails of diabetics.

Gout

Gout is another metabolic disease with a particular predilection for the feet. In gout, the body either overproduces or underexcretes a substance known as uric acid which eventually precipitates as sodium urate crystals which become deposited in the feet, mostly in the big toe joint. These deposits are known as tophi and will eventually destroy the toe joint. Gout can also affect other parts of the body such as the heel, the hands and even the ear lobes.

Gout attacks are sudden and excruciatingly painful. The pain is often described as "pulsating" or "crushing" and can be so severe that even the weight of a bed sheet on the foot can be agonizing. The gouty joint becomes red and swollen and feels hot to the touch.

Gout is generally hereditary and occurs most often in heavy middle-aged men. Benjamin Franklin was known to have suffered from it. Gout can be related to diet. Foods such as sardines, anchovies, liver, and sweetbreads contain a high concentration of purines, a type of protein. When purine rich foods are broken down uric acid concentration rises. Gout has often been referred to as the rich man's disease, but the poor are not exempt. It's rich food—not money in the bank—that aggravates this condition.

Alcohol consumption is also associated with gouty attacks because it decreases the body's excretion of uric acid. The classic gout attacks occur shortly after one has consumed much food and liquor at a party. Activities involving exercise or stress also seem to evoke gouty attacks.

After the attack has passed, a gout afflicted patient will generally be free of symptoms. This sometimes lulls one into believing that he is cured. Unfortunately, such is not the case. Months or even years later another gout attack will occur and after that will reappear at more frequent intervals.

Gout can also occur as a result of other diseases or medicines taken. The popular diuretics Diuril® (chlorothiazide) and Hydrodiuril® (hydrochlorothiazide) tend to elevate uric acid levels and have been known to precipitate an attack. Insulin, penicillin, aspirin and ACTH can also be responsible.

Any disease which results in protein breakdown can similarly cause gout. Psoriasis, leukemia, and anemia are among the most common diseases in which secondary gout is found.

Prevention

Once you have been diagnosed as having gout, you can prevent or minimize attacks as follows:

1. Stay on a low purine diet consisting of foods such as vegetables, cheeses, eggs, fruits, milk and cereal. Avoid meats and fish whenever possible.

2. Minimize alcohol consumption.

3. Take your prescribed medicine every day. Your physician may place you on a drug which inhibits uric acid formation such as Zyloprim® (allopurinol). It is essential that you continue this drug, even if you have not had a gout attack recently. If you

discontinue taking your medicine, you leave yourself vulnerable to another gout attack.

Treatment

The treatment for an acute gout attack of the foot is as dramatic as the attack itself. A podiatrist or physician injects a small amount of local anesthetic into the nerve innervating the big toe joint, which immediately relieves the pain. This so-called "nerve block" also causes a large increase in the blood flow to the big toe which redissolves the sodium urate crystals deposited there. Your physician may follow up this injection with a prescription of an anti-inflammatory medication such as Butazolidin Alka® (phenylbutazone).

This method of treatment is generally superior to the old standard treatment of hourly doses of colchicine, a medication which often caused nausea, vomiting, and diarrhea.

Vascular Diseases

The arteries and veins in the feet are the smallest and farthest away from the heart and are therefore among the first to be affected by any vascular disease. Arteriosclerosis (hardening of the arteries), for example, can be detected very early by palpating the pulses in the feet.

Raynaud's Disease

In Raynaud's disease, the small arteries of both the toes and the fingers go into spasm when exposed to the cold. This causes the fingers and toes to exhibit a classic color change sequence from white to blue to red. Raynaud's attacks can also be brought on by increased emotional stress. These attacks are quite painful but will gradually subside over the course of time. Raynaud's attacks are best prevented by the elimination of emotional stress and by wearing warm protective socks and gloves when exposed to cold weather. Vasodilating drugs may be useful as would be the drinking of a small amount of alcohol.

Acrocyanosis is another vascular disease which mimics Raynaud's disease. In this condition, the toes (and sometimes the fingers) turn blue. This blueness is painless and often brought on by cigarette smoking, which causes the arteries to constrict. The cessation of smoking usually resolves this condition.

Erythromelalgia is a circulatory condition which is almost the antithesis of Raynaud's disease and acrocyanosis. A patient with erthromelalgia finds that his feet may become so unbearably hot that he must soak them in ice water or sleep with feet extending out from his bed. The treatment for this condition consists of taking vasoconstricting medications such as ergotamine. Oddly enough, erthyromelalgia is one condition which may actually be *helped* by the smoking of cigarettes (again because it constricts blood vessels)!

A more complete discussion of arterial and venous diseases can be found in the next chapter.

The Aging Foot 10

No segment of our population is more sensitive to the importance of the feet than the elderly. Our society puts a premium on the ability to "get around." If you lose that ability, you will greatly limit the number of activities you can participate in, and you will also lose much of your body's defensive capability. As muscle tone deteriorates, so does circulation. This means that maintaining good foot health can increase your lifespan. Being an invalid can be psychologically debilitating to anyone—but to an older person who has been independent all his life, it is an especially devastating blow.

A reduced birth rate and new advances in medicine have led to a greater proportion of old people in our society today. But the expression, "you're only as young as you feel" is as true as ever. The American Podiatry Association recently produced a film and an accompanying booklet entitled "You're Only as Young as Your Feet." Awkward, painful walking can add years to your appearance. An individual's gait is often one of the first things you notice. Your footsteps identify you. Are you making a youthful impression?

Foot problems are much more common in the elderly than in the general population. Bad feet do not develop overnight. Conditions such as bunions, hammertoes, corns, arthritis, and arteriosclerosis (hardening of the arteries) can take years to develop and they tend to get worse with time. The older you are, the greater your chances of developing a foot problem.

Arthritis of the Foot

Perhaps the most common malady affecting the aging foot is osteoarthritis, a type of arthritis resulting from the chronic wear of bones and joints. The bones and joints of the foot support more weight than any other part of the body and unfortunately the hundreds of thousands of miles of walking we have logged by the time we become senior citizens make osteoarthritis an almost inevitable prospect for our later years. Heavy individuals are especially prone to this form of arthritis.

The symptoms of osteoarthritis follow a classic pattern. Early in the morning your affected joints are stiff and painful. After some walking, the stiffness gradually diminishes, only to return later in the day and become progressively worse by evening.

The foot joints most subject to osteoarthritis are the metatarsal joints (at the ball of your feet). These joints assume the most force during walking. A bunion is a dramatic form of osteoarthritis which occurs at the first metatarsal-phalangeal joint. A bunion is characterized by a large accumulation of extra bone behind the big toe on the inside border of the foot. In a severe bunion the big toe drifts laterally (toward the outside of the foot), sometimes overlapping or underlapping the second toe. As the big toe drifts over, the metatarsal joints are gradually destroyed. The end product is a painful, ugly-looking foot which will not fit comfortably into conventional shoes.

The toes are also affected by osteoarthritis. A hammertoe results from the "buckling up" of the small joints of the toes. A thickening of these joints often results at the knuckles (proximal interphalanageal joints). The raised position of a hammertoe predisposes the formation of corns. The top of the toe rubs against the top of the shoe, irritating the skin and stimulating the growth of a corn.

Rheumatoid Arthritis

Rheumatoid arthritis is a more destructive and disabling arthritis which generally begins much earlier in life. Most commonly affected are females in their twenties and thirties. The exact cause of this progressive disease is unknown, but we do know that it is aggravated by physical and emotional stress and most often affects both the ankles and the small joints of the toes symmetrically.

Management

If you suffer from either form of arthritis, your most immediate goals are elimination of pain and maintaining the range of motion of your joints. These usually go hand in hand. The pain/ motion cycle develops as follows: pain in the joints causes a limitation of motion of the joints which in turn leads to more pain and so on. Breaking the pain cycle leads to more motion, which in turn leads to less pain and so on.

Analgesic and anti-inflammatory drugs are useful in decreasing pain. The most cost-effective of these are the non-steroidal salicylates. Ordinary aspirin is still one of the safest, most effective medicines available for the treatment of arthritis. Each year another new "miracle" drug is introduced. Motrin®, Indocin®, and Clinoril®, among others, have all at one time held the limelight. The newest touted drug at this writing is Feldene®. Your podiatrist or rheumatologist will prescribe his favorite anti-arthritic drug. You may have to try a few of these drugs until you find the one that is the most effective and has the fewest side effects.

If a joint in your foot is acutely painful, it may require an injection of a steroid mixed with a local anesthetic. The local anesthetic immediately numbs the joint and allows you to walk normally. This breaks up adhesions and allows the joint to regain its normal range of motion. The steroid acts as an anti-inflammatory agent to help maintain the joint in a non-irritated state.

Physical therapy is a highly recommended adjunct to any arthritic treatment program. The age-old remedy of soaking your feet in warm water and epsom salts is a very effective method of "loosening up" your joints. After you have soaked for about fifteen minutes, begin to manipulate your toes. Start by gently pulling out on the toes. This opens up the joint spaces. Next, while maintaining some outward pulling force on the joint, begin to move the toe up and down through its available range of motion. Move the toe only as far as it will comfortably go. *Do not force it!*

After you have manipulated each toe, dry your feet and take a short walk. You'll be surprised how good your feet will feel.

You may want to use a whirlpool instead of a tub to soak your feet in. The best whirlpools are those that vigorously force a stream of water toward your feet. Jacuzzi® and Pollenex® are two brands that have this feature. Avoid the type of foot baths that merely agitate the water—they're only slightly more effective than a plain tub of water.

If you do not get sufficient relief from a whirlpool, see your physical therapist or podiatrist. He is likely to have more sophisticated equipment such as ultrasound or electro-galvanic stimulators. These modalities are able to penetrate much deeper than a whirlpool and provide more relief to your joints.

Walking forces the joints of the feet to remain active and is thus a vital part of any arthritic treatment program. You should aim to walk a reasonable amount each day. Depending on the severity of your arthritis, this could range from a few blocks to a few miles. Whatever your limits, make the effort—you'll feel better for it.

Circulatory Disorders

The blood vessels supplying the feet are the farthest away from the heart. They are also the smallest and thus the first to react to any disease which affects the circulation. Arterial disorders such as arteriosclerosis and diabetes often produce their first symptoms or signs in the feet.

The venous system of the foot and the lower leg are also subject to particular strain. Once your blood has reached your feet, it must rise upward against the force of gravity. Venous disorders such as varicose veins and thrombophlebitis occur exclusively in the leg and ankle area.

The swollen ankles experienced by many senior citizens are often a result of the inability of the veins to perform their job of returning blood to the heart. Swollen ankles can also serve as an "early warning" detector for major systemic disorders such as congestive heart failure, kidney or liver disease. If your ankles are swollen, see your doctor.

Arterial Disease

Do your feet often feel cold? Have you lost hair from your legs or the top of your feet? Are your nails thickened? Does pain force you to stop walking every few blocks or after climbing a few stairs? Do you wake up in the middle of the night with cramps?

While in the sitting position, check the color of your feet. Do they look reddish or bluish? Now raise your feet to a level above your heart. Do they now look pale or whitish?

These are all classic signs and symptoms of vascular disease, the most common of which is arteriosclerosis. This is a slowly developing disorder in which cholesterol-containing fatty plaques accumulate on the inside of the vessels. These deposits decrease the inside diameter of the artery and thus reduce blood flow to the feet.

Loss of hair, thickening of the nails and cold feet are early signs of decreased blood flow. As arterial disease progresses, pain will result from any activity which requires more blood flow. This pain, known as intermittent claudication, will force you to stop after walking a certain number of blocks or climbing flights of stairs. As the disease progresses, the amount of activity you can perform will decrease. Patients complain, "Last year, I had to stop walking every six blocks. This year I have to stop every four blocks."

Eventually the disease may become so severe that pain is present even at rest. This "rest pain" occurs most often in the middle of the night.

Healthy feet have a pinkish hue regardless of position. Feet with poor circulation may look normal in the lying down position, but if you dangle them for a few minutes they will assume a reddish or bluish tint. This occurs because the blood going to the foot is traveling so slowly that your body uses up most of the oxygen in it. If you elevate feet with poor circulation, they will appear blanched. This results from the inability of blood to overcome gravity and rise to the feet.

Prevention

There has been much speculation about the prevention of arteriosclerosis, but there is still a great deal that only research can tell us. Examination of the arteries of young American soldiers killed in the Korean War revealed the presence of deposits within their arteries which were previously thought to occur much later in life. This discovery opened up the whole question of the influence of diet on the development of arterial disease.

Diet

We know that obese individuals and those with diets rich in saturated fats and cholesterol have a high incidence of arterial disease. The question of cause and effect, though, remains controversial. While many experts recommend a lower intake of saturated fats and cholesterol to prevent arterial disease, other experts claim that dietary changes, particularly for the elderly, are of little or no value.

Common sense dictates moderation in your diet. The *total* amount of food you consume is probably more important than the specific amount of any one component. Few will dispute that a light to average weight individual stands a better chance of avoiding vascular disease.

Exercise

The role of exercise in preventing the development of arterial disease is better documented and less controversial than that of diet. During vigorous exercise the body releases *high-density lipoproteins* (HDLs). These HDLs act like detergents to chemically "clean and scrub" the inside of your vessels. HDLs *cannot* be bought at your local health food store—exercising is the only way to produce them.

While most senior citizens cannot be expected to train for marathons (although some do), it is important to begin regular "workouts"—whether it is a daily swim, a round of golf, some bicycling, or perhaps the most popular and easiest exercise of all, walking.

Walking

Evidence shows that brisk walking—from a hike in the wilderness to competitive racewalking—is nearly as good a fitness builder as running. President Harry Truman was an advocate of brisk early morning walks, convinced that they would help him live longer. Truman lived to age 88. Whatever route you choose, check with your physician first and then make it a part of your daily regimen. Ideally, you should start your program slowly and aim for from three to five half-hour workouts each week. Proper exercise will make you feel younger and healthier and may in the end be more important to your circulation than any medicine or dietary change.

Treatment

The treatment of arterial disease is aimed at insuring the maximum blood flow to the feet. Without sufficient blood flow, any injury to the foot cannot heal properly, and a small wound or ingrown toenail may lead to gangrene, resulting either in amputation or death. This happens all too often, particularly in those who suffer both arteriosclerosis and diabetes.

Pharmaceuticals

Unfortunately, medicines have little effect on diseased arteries. Most of these drugs are smooth muscle relaxers known as vasodilators. In theory they increase blood flow by allowing the thin layer of muscle in your arteries to expand. These expanded arteries are capable of carrying more blood. Ironically, these vasodilators (Vasodilan®, Cyclospasmol®, Nicobid®) work best in patients who have normal vessels and thus don't need them. The diseased vessels of those who could benefit from these drugs are often so hard that they simply cannot expand. Still, it may be worthwhile giving these drugs a try.

Surgery

In cases where the major arteries to the foot are blocked, bypass surgery may be indicated. In this type of surgery either a superficial vein or artificial graft is connected from a large open artery in your thigh to one in your foot or leg. This is complicated and somewhat risky surgery, but is often necessary to save a foot or leg.

A less dramatic and sometimes useful procedure attempts to relax the muscles in your arteries by cutting the nervous system's innervation to them. This attempt at "surgical vasodilation" is known as sympathectomy. This procedure has many of the limitations of chemical vasodilation (rigid vessels cannot expand), but may be of value in individual cases. Both sympathectomy and bypass should be performed only after careful evaluation by a peripheral vascular specialist.

Elevation/Dependency Exercises

If you are not capable of embarking upon a vigorous exercise program, you may still benefit from elevation/dependency exercises. Start by dangling your feet for a few minutes. Next, elevate your feet above the level of your heart for a few more minutes. Afterward, dangle your feet again and repeat the cycle. Performing this series of exercises several times a day will help you maintain your circulation.

Varicose Veins

Your veins have the difficult job of returning your blood, against gravity, to your heart. The body has many ways to assist in this action. When your calf muscles contract during walking, for instance, they help squeeze blood upward. "One-way" valves in your veins also prevent blood from flowing down.

As we get older, however, these valves may become less efficient. The result may be venous insufficiency manifested in varicose veins or swollen ankles. Although varicose veins are thought of mostly for their cosmetic unattractiveness, they present a serious risk to seniors. A varicose vein which is accidentally cut will bleed profusely. What would you do to stop the bleeding? If you only apply a pressure dressing, the bleeding may not stop! The correct treatment is to first *elevate* the leg, then, while it is elevated, apply pressure with a bandage.

Varicose veins can also result in painful ulcerations of the leg and ankle. These ulcerations are generally the end product of a progressive disease process which first causes the skin of the lower leg to become thickened and discolored. This "bark-like" skin is often itchy. Ulcers usually develop on the lower inside aspect of the leg, at the point where the venous pressure is the greatest.

Management

Standing still for long periods of time tends to aggravate venous conditions so . . .

1. Whenever possible try to raise your feet onto a footrest or chair.

2. Elevate the base of your bed by placing an encyclopedia or large telephone book under the end of your mattress.

3. Elastic stockings are useful in both the prevention and treatment of venous disorders. The most effective stockings are the custom-made type such as Jobst®. Pre-cut stockings, such as Sigvaris®, may be almost as good for average shaped legs.

4. Do not use heating pads or whirlpools.

Treatment

Varicose veins or ulcers which do not respond to conservative management will require the treatment of a peripheral vascular specialist. The surgical treatment of choice may be a procedure known as venous stripping. In this operation, the surgeon completely removes the incompetent vein(s) from your leg. A new and less radical non-surgical cure holds great promise for varicose vein sufferers. This procedure is known as "injection-compression sclerotherapy." Manhattan vein specialist Dr. Ken Biegeleisen contends that this procedure has been performed successfully in Europe for many years and can be performed safely in a doctor's office. A physician injects a solution into the incompetent vein which causes it to close up. An elastic compression bandage is then applied and worn for several weeks.

Phlebitis

Phlebitis is an inflammation of a vein which can result from injury, disease, (e.g., cancer), or most frequently from unknown causes. The single most common predisposing factor is any debilitating illness which necessitates prolonged bedrest. If the leg is not exercised, the blood flow stagnates, and phlebitis may ensue.

There are two types of phlebitis. Superficial phlebitis occurs almost exclusively in varicose veins. This condition is rarely dangerous, although it can cause considerable pain for a week or two. The treatment for superficial phlebitis is an ace bandage and *walking*. Bed rest does not help—and it may in fact make things worse.

Deep vein phlebitis occurs in the major deep veins of the calf and thigh. This is a serious disease which can cause permanent swelling of the leg, and even death. The danger is that a large blood clot can break off and travel to the lung. Deep vein phlebitis does not grow out of the superficial variety; it is a distinct disease, requiring hospitalization and the use of chemical blood thinners.

Aging Skin

As you grow older, the activity of your oil producing glands decreases, causing your skin to become dry. The skin of the feet is particularly vulnerable to dryness. Our hands are constantly visible, so we tend to apply moisturing creams to them when we notice they look dry. But our feet, hidden under shoes and socks, are less accessible and are, as a result, too often ignored.

Take a good look at your feet. Is the skin moist looking or is it dry and scaly? Dry skin makes you look older. It also increases your chance of developing a foot infection. Dry skin has less strength than moist skin, so it runs an increased risk of cracking. Bacteria are always present on the outside of your skin and can enter your body through cracked skin.

Prevention and Treatment

Keeping your feet supple requires regular care. Get into the habit of applying a good moisturizing agent to your feet every day. It need not be an expensive cream—ordinary vegetable shortening such as Crisco® is fine. And if you are using a hand cream or lotion for your face or hands, you may certainly use it on your feet. The most effective way to use a moisturizer is to apply it after you have soaked your foot. This way, the cream acts to seal in the moisture that our skin has absorbed.

Thickened Nails

Your nails will generally thicken with age. This could be due to fungal infection, decreased circulation, or accumulated trauma to the nails. Thickened nails are unattractive and may cause a shoe fitting problem. Pain may result when the thickened nail presses against the top of the shoes.

Treatment

Thickened nails require the care of a podiatrist since using a standard clipper is nearly impossible. A podiatrist will use a high speed drill to grind the nail. Periodic visits to your foot doctor will keep your nails looking as normal as possible.

Foot Surgery   11

Foot surgery has undergone tremendous changes in the past few decades. In the first half of the twentieth century the emphasis was on correcting the physical manifestation of the problem with little effort made toward addressing the forces behind the deformity—in much the same manner that a mechanic may replace a tire with uneven wear without realigning the wheels. This tendency contributed to unacceptably high failure and recurrence rates in foot care. Also a factor was the lack of sophisticated instruments available. As recently as 1970 many surgeons were still utilizing modified hammers and chisels to perform foot surgery. Today, most foot surgery is performed with high-speed power equipment that enables the surgeon to make precise bone incisions.

Today's foot surgery focuses on getting the patient walking as soon as possible, sometimes immediately after surgery. This is in sharp contrast to foot surgery of the past, which too often left the patient immobilized for long periods of time. Still, the decision to have foot surgery is not one to be taken lightly. If you are considering having foot surgery, keep the following information in mind:

1. *Almost all foot surgery is elective.* You should have your foot operated on only after you have tried more conservative therapies. A heel spur, for example, will often respond to strapping, steroid injections or to the wearing of orthotic devices (customized sole inserts), so you owe it to yourself to try these

therapies first. Do what is best for *you*, not what is most expedient for the *surgeon*.

However, in the case of certain conditions, such as painful bunions or hammertoes, the conservative option, such as wearing a molded shoe, may be unacceptable to you. If this is the case, surgery may be the only alternative.

2. *Avoid "same day" surgery.* Most foot conditions develop slowly. This gives you the time to make a careful, sound decision. Don't let yourself be pressured while you're "in the chair." If you have doubts, go home and sleep on it. You may also want to get a second opinion. Most health insurance companies will be more than happy to send you to a qualified doctor, often at no charge to you.

The *only* type of surgery that should be performed during your first visit is minor skin surgery—such as the removal of an infected ingrown toe nail or the removal of a skin tumor such as a wart.

Occasionally emergency surgery is necessary, as in the diagnosis of osteomyelitis (bone infection) but this is a rare occurence. There is no valid reason why corrective bone surgery can't be scheduled at your convenience.

3. *Elect a time that is best for you.* Since foot surgery is elective, plan to have it done when you will be least inconvenienced. Swelling results from most foot surgery and necessitates the wearing of a surgical shoe for a few weeks. If you have to attend a wedding, you'll probably want to delay the procedure until after the festivities. If your job requires the wearing of stylish shoes, you may want to delay the surgery until your vacation.

Weather may also be a factor in the choice of your surgery date. Most people who live in a cold climate prefer to have their feet operated on in warmer weather because it is easier to fit a swollen foot into a sandal than a winter boot.

4. *Cosmetics alone is not a good reason to have foot surgery.* You may consider your foot problem unattractive but, unless you model your feet for a living, it's usually best to leave them alone. Good reasons for having foot surgery are to relieve pain, to help you walk better, or to help you fit into normal shoes.

5. *Select the best foot surgeon available.* Find out the qualifications of your surgeon. Every podiatrist or orthopedist is legally permitted to operate on your feet, but the training and experience of

individuals varies widely. While there is no one criterion by which to judge an individual's competence, you should look for the following attributes: a) completion of a surgical residency; b) board certification; c) hospital surgical privileges; d) satisfied patients; and e) a good reputation among other specialists.

A doctor who over-advertises to obtain surgical patients should be considered suspect—a top foot surgeon needs only his track record as his advertisement. Your surgeon should not be offended if you ask for a second opinion or a copy of your X-rays.

There are first-rate surgeons in every large city, so invest the time and energy to seek these individuals out. You deserve the best.

6. *Foot surgery is not painful.* Many procedures can be performed under local anesthesia. Your foot can be numbed with a Novocaine-like substance. Marcaine® is popularly used because it keeps the foot pain-free for about twelve hours. More extensive foot surgery is usually done under general anesthesia.

If you are in pain after the anesthetic wears off, many analgesic tablets, ranging from aspirin to narcotics are available to keep you pain free.

7. *Allow time for your foot to heal.* Modern surgical techniques now allow you to walk on an operated foot shortly after surgery. But don't expect to be running a marathon the following week. Nature needs time to fully heal the foot and this can vary with the individual. Some "fast healers" return to work a few days after surgery. Others need a week or more to recover. The duration and extent of the surgery are also factors. In general, the more extensive the surgery, the longer the recovery time.

The foot's healing process occurs in two stages. In the first phase, known as the "primary" healing stage, the body actively heals the incisions. This period lasts three to four weeks and you will be aware of the process.

In the "secondary" healing stage, your body gradually remodels the bones which have been operated on. This stage can take from several months to several years, and you will rarely be aware of the underlying changes. Gradually you will be able to resume all normal activities but you may occasionally feel a funny numbness, twinge, tingling or other sensation. When these disappear you know that the healing process is complete.

Office Versus Hospital Surgery

Where to have your surgery is an often controversial subject. Simply put, minor foot surgery should be performed in a doctor's office and major foot surgery should be performed in a hospital. But there are complicating factors. Some surgeons offices now contain operating suites as elaborate and well prepared as those in hospitals. And some procedures previously thought of as being major are now considered minor. So, where your procedure should be done depends ultimately on how much support care you need. Most doctors' offices are not equipped for such ancillary services as general anesthesia, attending physicians or nursing. Nor are they equipped for overnight stays. If your surgery is extensive, if you have a medical problem, such as a heart condition, or if you have no one to care for you at home, you will be better off in a hospital. If your procedure is minor, you are in good health and have someone to take care of you at home, you're better off having your surgery performed in a well-equipped doctor's office.

Conventional versus Minimal Incision Surgery

Two distinct techniques of foot surgery are currently being utilized and there is a great deal of controversy over the advantages and disadvantages of each method.

Conventional foot surgery is the predominant style used by hospital based surgeons. In this technique, the surgeon makes a lengthy incision over the area to be operated on and proceeds to "open up" the area. The surgeon can then visualize the internal structures and proceeds to cut and "remodel" bone using power drills and saws. Scalpel blades are often used to cut and reposition soft tissue structures such as tendons and capsules. This type of surgery is often referred to as "open" surgery.

Minimal incision surgery is performed predominantly in doctors' offices. In this technique a small incision is made over the involved area. A small dental-type drill is used to "grind off" bone. This method is often referred to as "closed" surgery since the surgeon cannot visualize the actual bone.

It is this inability to literally see the bone which fuels the vigorous opposition of many surgeons to "closed" surgery. They argue that due to the comparatively "blind" technique many unidentified structures are cut. They also point out that often necessary ancillary procedures such as the insertion of a joint implant or repositioning of tendons and joint capsules are simply not possible with minimal incision surgery.

Minimal incision surgeons contend that their technique offers the following advantages:

1. It can be performed in a doctor's office, thus saving considerable expense to the patient.

2. The patient does not have to remain in the hospital overnight. He may immediately ambulate, and often return to work within days.

3. The scar is usually smaller.

Minimal incision surgeons also argue that with the use of X-rays during the actual surgery, they *do* know what structures they are cutting.

It is probable that advances in technology which will improve the ability of the "closed" surgeon to see the structures he is cutting will in turn enhance the scope and safety of procedures. The photon image intensifier, which acts like a portable fluoroscope to make the underlying bones "visible" is just one of the many devices holding such promise.

The technique performed on your foot will depend on both the training of your surgeon and the severity of your foot condition. Small procedures such as the elimination of bone spurs on the toes are most easily corrected by minimal incision surgery. Major foot deformities involving the replacement of joints can only be corrected using "open" techniques. There are some conditions such as metatarsal deformities and minor bunion operations in which either technique can be utilized.

Soft Tissue Procedures

These procedures do not involve the cutting of bone. They range from the simple removal of a wart to the more complicated removal of a deep nerve tumor (neuroma).

Wart Surgery

As discussed, warts are benign skin tumors caused by a virus infection. They are commonly found on the bottom surface (plantar) of the foot and therefore are usually referred to as "plantar warts." Technically warts are known as verrucae and papillomas. Surgical excision of a wart is indicated in cases when the growth is large or when non-surgical therapy such as the use of acid has not been successful.

The surgeon first applies local anesthesia to numb the wart area and then uses an instrument known as a curette to "scoop out" the entire growth. No sutures (stitches) are needed to close the wound and usually no significant scar results. Sometimes a cauterizing agent such as phenol is used to help prevent the wart from recurring.

This procedure is not debilitating. The area where the procedure was performed may feel sore for a few days, and there may be some bleeding, but you should be able to return to your job the next day.

Nail Surgery

Nail surgery is also a relatively minor procedure. The most common indications are chronically ingrown and infected nails, in which case a small section of the side of the nail is usually removed. If you have a history of repeated infections of the same nail, the growth portions (nail root and matrix) at the back of the nail may also be removed. This can be accomplished by surgically removing these "growing" sections. More commonly, a caustic phenol solution is applied to these areas to prevent regrowth. The result is that the major portion of the normal nail will continue to grow, while the offending ingrown section will not. This procedure is both simple and highly effective. Occasionally, however, the offending portion of nail will regrow and the procedure will have to be repeated.

In some cases of severely deformed or fungus-infected nails, it may be necessary to remove the entire nail. Again, you and your doctor will make the decision as to whether this procedure should be temporary or permanent (removal of the entire growth plate). Permanent removal of a nail is not as drastic as it sounds. Your toenails serve little function and you can do very well without them. After this procedure is performed, a "nail-like" tough skin forms where the nail originally was. This can be covered with nail polish or an artificial nail.

Removal of a nail portion is not debilitating. You may, however, have to wear loose-fitting shoes for a few days after the procedure.

Morton's Neuroma

Morton's neuroma is a fairly common benign nerve growth usually developing between the third and fourth metatarsals and most often found in women. It is caused by the irritation of branches of the medial and lateral plantar nerve as they cross between the metatarsal bones.

Wearing tight shoes pushes the metatarsals together, squeezing the tumor between them, and this friction causes the nerve to enlarge. Symptoms of a neuroma vary but may include a sharp, tingling or burning sensation that radiates to the toes.

The conservative treatment of a neuroma includes injections of steroid into the neuroma as well as changing to wider shoes. If these measures are not successful, surgery may be necessary.

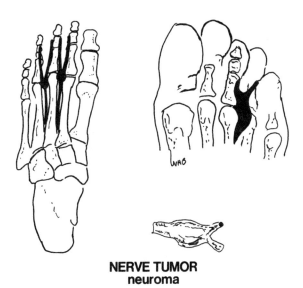

NERVE TUMOR
neuroma

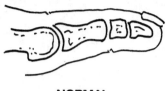

NORMAL

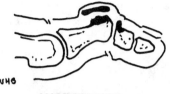

HAMMER TOE
with bone deformity

The procedure for neuroma removal requires an incision over the neuroma site. The surgeon then must carefully dissect and remove the entire tumor. Often the ligaments attaching the adjoining metatarsals are cut. This allows these metatarsals to separate and helps prevent recurrence of the tumor. Neuroma removal can be performed in either an office or hospital. This procedure requires sutures and you will have to wear loose shoes or sandals for about two weeks afterward.

Toe Procedures

Most toe procedures are designed to eliminate painful corns. These accumulations of extra skin develop because of excessive friction on the skin of the toe as it gets pressed between the bone on the inside and the shoe on the outside. This is usually caused

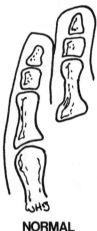

NORMAL

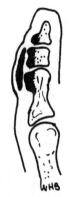

HARD CORN
with bone deformity

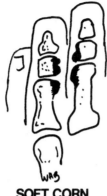

SOFT CORN
with bone deformity

by two structural conditions: most commonly, the tendons of the toe gradually contract causing the toe to "buckle up" and rise. As the "knuckle" of the toe rises higher, it is likely to rub against the top of the shoe, thereby causing a corn. When this condition occurs at the middle of a toe it is known as a *hammer-toe*. *Mallet toe* results when the buckling occurs at the end of the toe.

The second condition which may cause a corn is the presence of a bone spur on a toe. A bone spur—technically known as an "exostosis"—is a calcium deposit which forms on an area of bone subject to great friction. Bone spurs usually form at the ends and the sides of toes. The most common location for this type of corn is on the outside of the little toe, where friction against tight shoes is the greatest.

Corns due to bone spurs can also occur in between the toes as the skin gets rubbed between two toe bones. These corns be-

SUBUNGUAL EXOSTOSIS

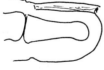

normal bone   **overgrowth of bone**

come soft and rubbery due to the presence of moisture between the toes and are known as "soft" corns. Another place that corns caused by bone spurs are likely to occur is at the end of a toe. Occasionally these bone spurs occur underneath a nail causing a painful condition known as a *subungual exostosis*.

"Soft Tissue" Toe Surgery—Tenotomy

A tenotomy is a simple procedure available for the correction of a hammertoe. Tenotomies are useful only in hammertoe cases where the problem is being caused by a contracted (tightened) tendon. The tendons going to your toes are located just below the skin. Look down at the top of your foot. If your tendons are tight, you can probably see them as "cord-like" structures. In a tenotomy, the surgeon uses a tiny blade to sever a tight tendon on the top of your foot, beyond your toes. Occasionally the tendon on the bottom of the toe is also cut. Sometimes the surgeon will also perform a capsulotomy in which he cuts the joint capsule just below the tendon as well.

Tenotomies are only useful when a hammertoe deformity is "flexible." By "flexible," we mean that the toe can be manually straightened. When a hammertoe has progressed to the point where the "knuckle" joint becomes rigid, a tenotomy to relax the tight tendon will be of little value. If you have a hammertoe, reach down and try to straighten the toe. If you can easily straighten the toe, a tenotomy may be indicated. If the toe is "stiff" and unbending, a tenotomy (or capsulotomy) by itself will be virtually useless. If your corn is a result of a bone spur, it is also unlikely that you will benefit from a tenotomy.

Perhaps the most compelling limitation to the tenotomy is that its benefits tend to be temporary. After the procedure you will need to stretch the corrected toe daily for many months to prevent the tendon from reshortening.

Bone Procedures for Toe Problems

The most effective long-term cures for corns due to hammertoes and bone spurs are procedures that either straighten the toe or remove the offending spur. When the corn occurs near the "knuckle" or joint, a procedure known as an arthroplasty is performed using either the open or closed technique. In the open method, an incision is made on the top of the toe and a section of bone at the raised area of the "knuckle" is removed. In the closed method, a small incision is made on the top or the side of the toe and a burr is inserted into the bone, and rotated by a dental-type drill. The excess bone is pulverized into bone paste which is then squeezed out of the small hole on the top of the toe. The advantage of the closed technique is that only a tiny scar will remain after the toe has healed. The advantage of the open method is that there is less chance of subsequent stiffening of the joint. In the open procedure, the offending bone is cleanly removed from the joint space. In the closed or minimal incision technique, bone paste can be left in the joint and this paste can regrow to form bone which may result in a stiff or arthritic joint. Each procedure takes about thirty minutes and can be performed in a doctor's office under local anesthesia. If you have this procedure done on a Friday, expect to be back to work on Monday (albeit in loose or cut-out shoes).

As in any procedure performed on the foot, it is important that no pressure be put on the operated area. Your doctor may give you wooden "post-op" shoes, or you may choose to wear loose-fitting sneakers or an old pair of shoes with a hole cut in the top. If the weather is warm, sandals are also acceptable. Whatever you select, remember that no pressure is to be put on the healing wound for several weeks.

Surgery for "Spurs" on Toes

Bone spurs are actually calcium deposits which result from increased pressure or friction on bone. The body "lays down" this calcium for protection in the same way that the skin develops callus to protect itself from excessive force. Technically known as an *exostosis*, this is basically a permanent condition which *cannot* be helped by reducing the amount of calcium in your diet.

Bone spurs can occur anywhere on your foot. You may be able to feel them as small lumps and bumps. Often these lumps are painless. If this is the case, leave them alone. Sometimes they may result in corns, particularly when they develop on the outside of the little toe or between the toes, where they result in "soft" corns. Surgery is indicated when you can no longer get relief from wider shoes.

A *subungual exostosis* occurs when a bone spur develops underneath a toenail. Surgery is indicated for this painful condition when you can no longer get relief from wearing a shoe with a higher toe box (the part of the shoe above the toes).

In the case of a simple exostosis, in which there is no joint involvement, closed surgery can be used to easily grind off the extra bone. This procedure is done in an office under local anesthesia and usually requires no sutures. An exostosis can also be removed via open surgery. Ultimately it is up to your surgeon to choose the method, but it is important for you to be aware of the options.

Metatarsal Surgery

The metatarsals are the "long" bones of your feet. The "ball" of the foot is the area located below the front part of the metatarsal bones. Metatarsal problems range from the bunion, which is the deformity occurring at the first metatarsal, to a "tailor's bunion" which is found on the fifth metatarsal. Plantar-flexed or "dropped" metatarsals are a condition which often results in painful callus formation on the bottom of the foot.

Bunion Surgery

A bunion is a deformity found at the first metatarsal-phalangeal joint, behind your big toe. It is a condition that develops slowly and results from the gradual dislocation of the metatarsal-phalangeal joint which has become "unstable" during the propulsive phase of walking (a time when the joint *should* be stable). As the deformity progresses, the big toe itself will shift toward the outside of the foot. In severe cases, the big toe will actually overlap or underlap the second toe. Bunions are often painful and they can make shoe fitting very difficult. Contrary to what many people believe, tight shoes do not *cause* bunions, but they will aggravate them and accelerate their development. The tendency for bunion formation is hereditary and surgery is the only way to correct them. Exercises, splints, and other devices look good on paper but they just *don't work*. The forces causing a

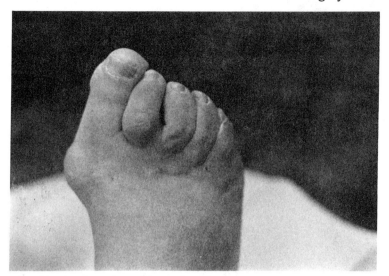

Typical bunion formation with associated hammertoes

bunion are simply too great for any known device to correct. Orthotics designed to stabilize the foot during gait are custom-made inserts which fit into your shoes. While these devices do not correct a bunion, they may be useful in providing relief and slowing down bunion development.

If your bunions don't hurt and you don't have difficulty finding shoes, there is no need for surgery. You should, however, see a podiatrist about having orthotics made to counteract de-

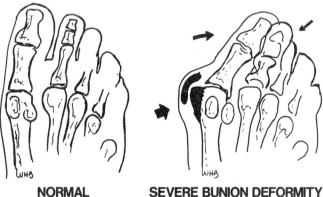

NORMAL   **SEVERE BUNION DEFORMITY**

forming foot forces. If your bunions are painful, bunion surgery is indicated.

Most of the recent advances in foot surgery have been directed at bunion surgery. In the past, emphasis was placed on the removal of the "exostosis" or lump, and straightening of the big toe. The reasoning was "if the toe looks straight, it will function properly." Each surgeon had his own favorite procedure. Today, we know that there are many different types of bunions and that no single procedure will give the best results. Your surgeon must first X-ray your foot to determine the type of joint you have. He will then measure the various angles of your foot. Only

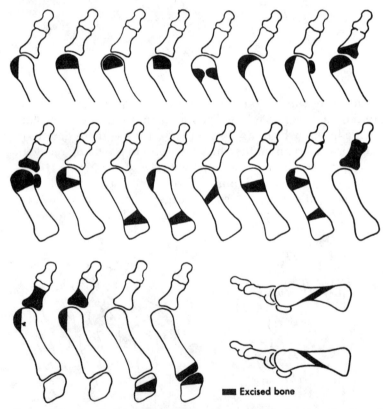

■ Excised bone

Some of the hundreds of different procedures available for the correction of bunion deformity (from DuVrie's Surgery of the Foot, *C.V. Mosby)*

then can he determine which procedure is best for your bunion. Procedure selection is very important. No matter how expertly the surgery is done, your results are only as good as the procedure selected.

In a "simple" bunion, where the toe is straight, only the exostosis need be removed. This procedure can be done either in an open or closed manner. Most bunions, however, are not simple and require either cutting of capsular tissue, or cutting of bone (osteotomy). These procedures are generally best done using the open technique, in which there is less chance of traumatizing the first metatarsal-phalangeal joint.

Depending on the nature and severity of the bunion, your surgeon and you will decide whether to perform the procedure in an office or hospital and whether to have the operation done under local or general anesthesia. If you have bunions on both feet, you'll want to decide whether or not to have them corrected at the same time. Each choice has its own advantages and disadvantages. You'll initially have a longer recuperation time when you have both feet operated on at the same time, but you may feel that this is preferable to having one foot operated on and then having to go back and do the other foot later.

The recovery period from bunion surgery will vary depending on the specific procedure and your body's healing rate. Most people can walk satisfactorily within a few days after surgery. Again, you will have to wear modified footgear until the post-op swelling subsides. Some people need a couple of months to return to normal shoes. Don't expect to be a "cripple" after bunion surgery, but don't expect to go dancing the week after either. If you work at a desk job, expect to return to work the week after surgery. If you have a walking job or have both feet operated on at the same time, your disability time will probably be two weeks or more. Keep in mind that these are general guidelines which your surgeon may modify. Don't be misled by advertisements for "lunch-hour" bunion surgery—you may turn out to be "the slowest healer" the doctor has ever had!

Prevention of Bunion Recurrence

After bunion surgery you must take measures to prevent the recurrence of this deformity. The best way to do this is with orthotic devices, which act to control the faulty biomechanics responsible for the instability of the first M-P joint.

"Bunion-Like" Conditions

The joint involved in bunion formation (the first metatarsal-phalangeal or M-P joint) assumes more weight than any other foot joint in the propulsive phase of gait and is more likely to be affected by osteoarthritis, a condition resulting from excessive "wear and tear" in which extra bone is deposited near the joint. This extra bone restricts the motion of the joint and causes severe pain during walking.

While bunions result from a gradual dislocation of the joint, painful bunion-like conditions can occur in which there is no dislocation of the first M-P joint. In these cases, the big toe and joint will look straight, but will hurt when moved. In the early stages of osteoarthritis of the big toe joint, a small bone spur forms at the top or side of the joint. This spur causes a limitation of motion, creating a condition referred to as *hallux limitus*. If left untreated, eventually the condition progresses to the point where there is virtually no motion left in the joint. This is referred to as *hallux rigidus*.

The early stages of hallux limitus should be treated with physical therapy to maintain as much range of motion as possible. When normal ambulation is no longer possible, surgery is nec-

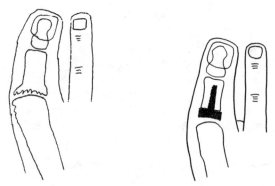

Surgical implant of Hallux Rigidus. On left note the ragged bone near the joint restricting motion. On right, an artificial implant restores motion to the joint.

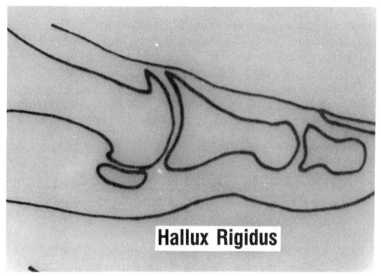

Note the bone spurs at the first metatarsal-phalangeal joint which restrict normal motion of this joint. This results in pain during walking.

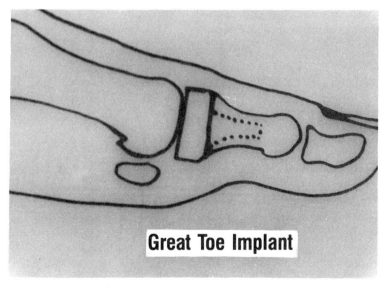

An inert silicon implant is used to replace a badly damaged arthritic joint.

essary to "remodel" the joint. This is an open procedure in which the excess bone surrounding the joint is excised and it is often necessary to replace the entire joint with an artificial implant. After this procedure it is important that vigorous physical therapy be instituted to maintain normal joint motion.

Osteoarthritis can also affect the lesser metatarsals. In these cases, therapy and treatment parallel that of osteoarthritis of the first M-P joint.

Tailor's Bunion

A tailor's bunion or "bunionette" is a bunion-like condition of the fifth M-P joint (the area behind the little toe). It derives its name from the old belief that tailors developed this condition as a result of working at their sewing machines with their legs crossed and the outside of their feet touching. This condition is caused by faulty foot mechanics and, like a conventional bunion, tends to be hereditary.

Two procedures are commonly used to correct the tailor's bunion. In some cases, an angulated incision is made in the bone, which is then slid inward. Other times the front or side part of the bone is removed. Regardless of which method is selected, this is generally a highly successful procedure, and post-op ambulation and healing are rapid.

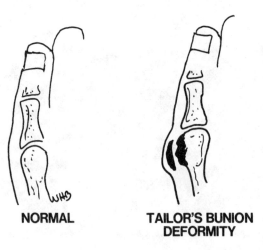

NORMAL   **TAILOR'S BUNION DEFORMITY**

Surgery for "Dropped" Metatarsals

Ideally, all five metatarsal bones should hit the ground at the same level. Often, however, one or more metatarsals can be structurally lower than the others. This condition is referred to as plantar-flexed or "dropped" metatarsals. The increased pressure of one metatarsal hitting the ground with more force than the others often results in the formation of a painful callus-like lesion known as an intractable plantar keratoma (IPK).

The conservative treatment of an IPK involves using an accom-

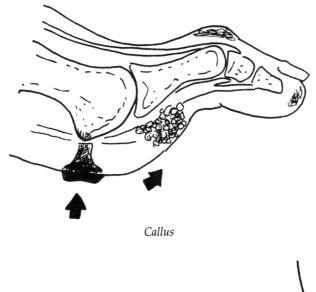

Callus

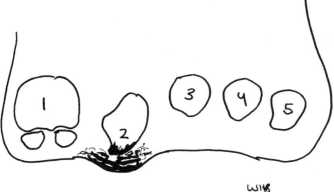

Intractable Plantar Keratoma (IPK)

modative orthotic with a built-in depression below the dropped metatarsal. While this device will not correct this condition, it will allow the dropped metatarsal to functionally hit the ground at the same level as the other metatarsals. In an older, less effective treatment, metatarsal pads were placed behind the affected bone. The theory was that these pads "raised" the dropped metatarsal. Experience has shown, however, that it is better to let a plantar-flexed metatarsal drop harmlessly into a small hole, than to attempt to "lift" it.

When conservative therapy has not been successful, surgery is indicated. This highly successful procedure, known as an *osteotomy* involves surgically raising the dropped metatarsal. This can be accomplished easily using either the open or closed method. In both cases, an incision is made into the metatarsal causing a precise surgical fracture. The patient is allowed to walk immediately in wooden post-op shoes which "float" the fractured bone and let it heal in a new raised position. Healing from an osteotomy takes about three weeks.

Heel Spur Surgery

A heel spur is a painful bone formation on the heel caused by the gradual "pulling off" of bone from the heel by the stretching of the ligaments of the arch. These ligaments originate in the heel and terminate in the metatarsal bones. Surgery is indicated only after all other conservative treatments have been unsatisfactory. For a detailed discussion of conservative therapy see page 83.

Heel spur surgery is performed through a small incision on the inside back part of the foot. It is no longer considered absolutely mandatory to remove the entire spur. Often detaching ligaments attaching to the spur (the plantar fascia) is sufficient to make this condition asymptomatic.

Major Foot Surgery

Major foot surgery is also available for the correction of foot deformities such as flatfeet, high arched feet, clubfoot, and ankle instability. Many of these procedures require the use of wires, screws and extensive casting to fixate bones. This type of surgery should therefore not be considered as "ambulatory." The procedures for these "reconstructive" surgeries are complex and are best discussed with your own surgeon.

What To Expect After Surgery

Foot surgery is unique—in what other type of surgery are you required to walk on a healing wound? The foot though, is a sturdy structure which responds well to this challenge, and most foot surgery heals uneventfully. But you should be prepared for any of the following possible post-op complications:

1. *Post-op swelling (edema)*. Some swelling should be expected following your operation. Generally, the more extensive the surgery, the greater the swelling will be. Elevating your feet will help reduce this swelling. One way you can do this is to place a large book such as an encyclopedia or Sears catalog under the base of your mattress. Remember that the more you're on your feet after surgery, the longer it will take for the swelling to go down. Most edema should be gone after one month. Some residual swelling, however, may remain for the next few months. This residual swelling should not be painful, but may restrict you from wearing tight-fitting shoes.

2. *Black and blueness*. This is a normal sequela of surgery and results from small internal bleeding in the wound site. Sometimes this discoloration may even appear in other parts of the foot. Bunion surgery, for example, might result in black and blue adjoining toes. Post-op discoloration will gradually fade and completely disappear within a month.

3. *Soreness*. This will also vary with the extent of surgery and your own pain threshold. Many people require little or no pain medication after surgery—often the application of ice is sufficient. Others use aspirin or Tylenol®. If you are in discomfort, your surgeon can prescribe medication ranging from codeine to stronger narcotics. Generally it makes sense to take as little medication as needed following surgery. Still, you don't have to be a hero. Take as much medicine as you need to feel comfortable. The soreness you feel after surgery will peak in about forty-eight hours and will decrease every subsequent day.

4. *Infections*. Your foot surgery was performed under sterile conditions, so the risks of infection are minimal. Keeping your bandages clean after surgery will also decrease the chances of an

infection developing, but unfortunately, even under the best of conditions infections may occur. Fortunately, modern antibiotics make infections much less of a problem than they once were. Be aware of the "cardinal" signs of an infection: throbbing pain, increased temperature, redness, swelling, pus.

Infections take a few days to develop. If you notice any of these signs, call your doctor immediately. The sooner an infection is detected, the faster it can be resolved.

5. *Numbness*. This is a normal post-operative finding that results from the cutting of small nerves during surgery. You may experience "funny" feelings such as a pins-and-needles sensation or an occasional sharp pain. These feelings are signs that your wound is healing and that the nerves are regenerating. Normal feeling should return to the operated part of your foot within a few months.

How To Choose a Podiatrist

12

The typical podiatrist is very competent and of high integrity. There are, however, podiatrists on both ends of the practice spectrum. Some are at the "top" of the profession with extraordinary expertise in such subspecialties as podiatric surgery, sports medicine, pediatrics, dermatology, rheumatology and peripheral vascular disease. By taking into consideration the following criteria, you will increase your chances of being treated by the most competent podiatrist available.

1. *American Podiatry Association membership.* A.P.A. membership is the first and most important standard in choosing a podiatrist. While membership does not insure skill, it does signify that the practitioner is bound to the ethical standards of the podiatry profession. Competency can be taught, ethics cannot. Members are affiliated through state podiatry societies. You may contact the A.P.A. directly by writing to 20 Chevy Chase Circle, N.W., Washington, D.C. 20015 or calling them at (202) 537-4900. A complete list of state societies is located on page 176.

2. *Referral from a friend or relative.* This is a valid way of helping you make a choice. If your friend or relative is satisfied with his current foot doctor, the probability is that you will be too. Do quiz your friend, however, on the specifics of the quality of the care. How complete was the examination? Did the doctor inquire about visits to other specialists? Did he seem concerned about your friend's health or did he seem rushed and disorganized?

151

Was your friend given alternatives for treatment or was he coerced into surgery that same day? Too often patients are influenced more by the doctor's personality than by the quality of care. So do question your friend thoroughly before following up with a visit.

3. *Physician referral.* Your family practitioner, internist, or pediatrician is a good source of referral. Establishment of a liaison between your podiatrist and physician benefits you by assuring ready consultation. Sending you to an incompetent doctor would reflect poorly on your physician, so he is putting himself on the line when he refers you to another specialist and you can feel reasonably secure with his choice.

4. *Hospital referral.* Your local hospital can refer you to a podiatrist who holds staff privileges. Hospitals tend to be very selective in their choice of staff. Hospital affiliation adds to a podiatrist's credentials, even if he does most of his surgery in the office.

5. *Board certifications.* This can be confusing. Some certifications are meaningful and some are not. All Doctors of Podiatric Medicine (D.P.M.) are "Diplomates" of the National Board of Podiatric Examiners. This designation only means that your podiatrist (as well as every other podiatrist) passed his board examinations *while in school.* The credentials of any podiatrist who lists this title are suspect. The only two valid certifying boards at this time are the American Board of Podiatric Surgery and the American Board of Podiatric Orthopedics. You may write to either of these boards at P.O. Box 31331, San Francisco, California, 94131 for a list of board certified podiatrists in your area.

6. *Specialty organizations.* It may be useful for you to find a podiatrist through a specialty organization. If you have a sports medicine problem you may contact the American Academy of Podiatric Sports Medicine. A list of foot surgeons operating through "conventional" incisions (open surgery) can be obtained by writing to the American College of Foot Surgeons. Both of these organizations share the same address: P.O. Box 31331, San Francisco, CA. 94131. For a list of surgeons operating through "minimal incisions" write to the American Academy of Ambulatory Foot Surgeons at Box 1976, Lynnwood, Washington 98036.

7. *Telephone directory.* This is a poor method of selecting *any* doctor. You are basically leaving your decision to chance. In general, if you have to choose a podiatrist by this method, do not be influenced by a large size listing. The quality of a podiatrist cannot be measured by the size of a listing. Nor can his skill be measured by the size of his practice. A poor practitioner with a good business sense can do quite well, at least for himself.

8. *Advertisements.* Solicitations for podiatry services either in newspapers or on radio and television are the poorest ways of selecting a podiatrist. Competent podiatrists do not need to advertise, and seldom do. *Beware* of advertisements which promise "free consultation" or "no out-of-pocket expenses." It is possible that you may wind up in a crowded, fast-paced office where you and your feet may be valued below the insurance payment the doctor will ask you to assign to him. You cannot expect quality foot care to be cheap. Choose a quality doctor and expect to assume at least part of the cost. Most ethical podiatrists will be willing to work out an acceptable payment plan with you.

The Profession of Podiatric Medicine

Podiatry is the medical specialty devoted to the diagnosis and treatment of foot disorders. Podiatrists are physicians of the foot trained in the medical and surgical alleviation and correction of foot problems.

Podiatry originated along with dermatology and dentistry as part of cosmetology, the external care of the body. Chiriatry (care of the hands) and podiatry (care of the feet) eventually became combined to form chiropody. This designation held until the twentieth century. The term chiropody has not been used in America for over thirty years, although it is still used in the United Kingdom.

The education and training of podiatrists has improved tremendously in the past thirty years. Today's podiatry student must meet the same entrance requirements as do traditional medical students, including taking the new MCATs. The first two years of podiatry schools are similar to traditional medical school and include such courses as anatomy, biochemistry, histology, microbiology, pathology, pharmacology, and radiology. The last two years consist of courses which specialize in the feet including foot surgery, biomechanics, podo-pediatrics, peripheral vascular disease and dermatology. These last two clinical years include externships in hospitals and clinics where the student receives hands-on training.

The graduating podiatrist receives the degree of Doctor of Podiatric Medicine (D.P.M) and then may choose a one, two or three year podiatric residency.

A Visit to Your Podiatrist—What to Expect

A visit to your foot doctor should be a pleasurable experience. In most cases, a podiatrist can provide you with immediate relief of pain. You should walk out of his office feeling better than when you came in.

Entering the office you will probably be met by a receptionist who will ask you to fill out an introductory form and may ask you some questions about your previous health history. Try to be as thorough as possible in answering these questions. The more information you provide the doctor, the easier it will be for him to make a proper diagnosis. You'll probably be asked about any medicines you may take, allergies you may have, and about previous surgery. Some patients ask, "What do these questions have to do with my feet? I only have a case of athlete's foot!" Your answers *are* important. The foot is not autonomous from the rest of the body. Your "athlete's foot" may in fact be a allergic reaction.

The more information you provide the doctor about your feet and the rest of your body, the better he will be able to diagnose and treat your condition. The pain in your big toe may be a manifestation of the metabolic disease known as gout. Often a podiatrist is the first to diagnose systemic diseases such as diabetes and congestive heart failure.

The Foot Exam

Once in the treatment room, expect a thorough examination of your feet. The doctor will do several tests to measure the circulation and neurological status of your foot. He will also take measurements for range of motion of your joints. If your problem is orthopedically related, he may ask you to walk, so that he can perform a gait analysis.

Do not be intimidated by the equipment in the office. Even the tub for a relaxing whirlpool can seem ominous. The drills a podiatrist uses to smooth down rough callus tissue might remind you of the dentist's, but will surprise you—they tickle rather than hurt. You may notice ultrasound machines and other physical therapy devices. These are used to help rehabilitate an injured foot or to help speed the healing of a foot which has recently been operated on. Ultrasound machines produce sound waves which are perceived as a warm comfortable feeling.

In most cases, you'll walk out of your podiatrist's office a lot more comfortable than when you came in.

X-Rays

X-rays can provide your doctor with important diagnostic information about your feet. They are however, never routine. If your doctor orders X-rays of your feet before he has even looked at them, find another doctor.

If you have a structural foot problem such as a corn due to a hammertoe or underlying bone spur, your podiatrist may need to take an X-ray of your foot. X-rays may also be necessary to locate a foreign body such as a pin or a piece of leaded glass.

Nobody likes X-rays. Fortunately, the X-ray machines used by most podiatrists are similar to the low dose machines used by dentists. The exposure you receive will be a small fraction of that from a large X-ray machine. It is still strongly recommended, though, that you insist on having a lead apron placed over your body.

A new type of X-ray machine known as a photon image intensifier requires no lead apron and may soon make conventional X-rays obsolete. These portable machines allow a doctor to instantly scan your bones in the same way that a fluoroscope is used. This allows the doctor to immediately determine if a bone is broken, for instance. There are no films to process. The photon image intensifier gives off approximately the same amount of radiation as your color television set.

Treatment

If your foot problem is minor, you may expect immediate treatment. This may consist of a prescription of a medicine, removal of corns or calluses, or removal of an ingrown nail. If more extensive treatment such as surgery is necessary, you will be told. Most foot surgery is elective and it is in your best interest to go home and "sleep on it." Foot surgery should be performed because *you* want it—knowing both the risks and benefits.

Same day surgery is not recommended, except for ingrown nail correction or the removal of a wart. In all other cases, you should arrange to have the procedure performed at your convenience. If you have any doubts as to the necessity of the procedure, seek out a second opinion. Many health insurance companies will arrange for this, often at no cost to you.

Fees

Your treatment plan should also include a frank discussion of fees. A podiatrist's fees are generally in line with other medical specialists. Most insurance plans include podiatry in their coverage. In some cases, such as with foot surgery, the doctor may accept part or all of your insurance as his payment. You should come to an understanding with your doctor as to what his fees are *before* you begin treatment. Do not hesitate to query the doctor, assistant, or receptionist about your financial responsibilities.

Footnotes

The following are some commonly asked questions about the feet. If you have any questions about the foot not covered in *Foot Talk*, send them to Dr. Block at 225 East 64th Street, New York, N.Y., 10021.

Is walking barefoot good for you?

A. Not particularly. Today's man-made surfaces present great hazards for your feet including stepping on broken glass, or getting a fungal infection or wart. Shoes are also necessary because man-made surfaces do not provide adequate shock absorption.

Naturalists often recommend that you walk on natural surfaces such as grass or sand. While these are somewhat safer than walking on man-made surfaces, the advantages of walking barefoot seem mostly hype. It was once pointed out to me that the famous Ethiopian marathoner Abebe Bikila had won the Olympic Gold Medal in Rome in 1960 while running barefoot. What was not mentioned was that when he won the gold medal in Tokyo four years later, he decided to wear sneakers.

What good if any does a whirlpool do for you?

A. A whirlpool was once the standard preliminary to any foot treatment. It has been abandoned by many podiatrists because it simply requires too much setting up. But whirlpools do serve a purpose: they soften and clean the skin and stimulate the circulation of the foot. But perhaps most importantly, soaking your feet in a whirlpool is a relaxing experience.

If you decide to buy a whirlpool for home use, select one which actively circulates a "jet stream" of water—some foot baths merely agitate the water. I recommend the Jacuzzi® and the Pollenex®.

What's the best thing to do for aching or tired feet?

A. Soaking in a whirlpool is a good start. You can also try the age-old remedy of soaking your feet in warm water and epsom salts—a few tablespoons will do.

Try to elevate your feet for a couple of minutes a few times a day. Sitting with your legs crossed at the ankle also helps them rest. If your feet ache constantly, see a podiatrist.

What's the difference between a chiropodist, a podiatrist and an orthopedic surgeon?

A. Chiropodists were the predecessors of today's podiatrists. Essentially they provided basic foot care. There are no chiropodists still practicing in America though the profession still exists in Great Britain, Australia and other countries.

A podiatrist is a physician licensed to diagnose and treat, both medically and surgically, any foot disorder. Podiatrists train for four years after college to earn the degree of Doctor of Podiatric Medicine (D.P.M.) One, two, and three year hospital residencies are available to podiatry school graduates.

An orthopedic surgeon is a specialist dealing with any bone deformity of the body. He first earns his medical degree in a traditional medical school. He then completes an internship and residency in orthopedic surgery. Some orthopedists specialize in deformities of the feet.

Both podiatrists and orthopedic surgeons perform foot surgery.

I saw an ad by a foot surgeon for microsurgery. What is this?

A. Microsurgery is a precise technique of operating under a microscope in which a surgeon can reattach tiny structures such as small blood vessels and veins. The most dramatic use of this technique is the reattachment of severed body parts such as fingers or toes.

Some surgeons who use minimal incision surgery (surgery done through small incisions), unethically misuse this term. True microsurgery is *not* indicated for the correction of such common foot conditions as hammertoes and bunions. If you require foot surgery and see an ad advertising microsurgery, you'll probably do better following the guidelines mentioned in Chapter 12.

I have diabetes. How often should I go to a podiatrist?

A. It depends on the type of diabetes you have and its severity. Juvenile diabetic patients should be checked every month by a podiatrist. Adult-onset diabetics can be seen at less frequent intervals, particularly if they are diet controlled.

Regardless of what type of diabetes you have, you should examine your feet daily. If you notice any signs of infection (redness, increase in temperature, swelling, pain, or the presence of pus) see your podiatrist immediately.

I noticed that my big toe is shorter than my second toe. I heard somewhere that this means I will have future foot problems. Is this true?

A. Not necessarily, but people with this condition, known as Morton's foot, do seem to have a higher incidence of foot problems. The big toe and its associated metatarsal are known as the first ray. This part of the foot is important in the propulsive stage of walking.

My feet are different sizes. How can I go about buying a pair of shoes that will fit properly?

A. As a general rule, you should always buy to fit the larger foot. This, however, will only help if your feet are almost the same size. If you wear totally different sizes, you should contact the National Odd Shoe Exchange. This is a nonprofit organization of over fifteen thousand members which arranges the exchange of odd size shoes among members. The address of this exchange is Rural Route 4, Indianola, Iowa 50125. Phone (515) 961-5125. Another possibility is to have custom molded shoes made.

What is laser surgery and how can it be used to help foot conditions?

A. A laser is an instrument which concentrates light into a powerful beam. This beam can be used to accurately cut tissue. Laser surgery has some distinct advantages over conventional surgery. The laser beam sterilizes, cauterizes (stops bleeding), and anaesthesizes as it cuts. The laser is also less traumatic to the tissue it cuts. This scalpel–less surgery is useful in the treatment of soft tissue tumors such as warts. Lasers can also be used for the surgical destruction of ingrown, malformed, or fungus infected nails.

At the present time, lasers cannot be used in bone surgery such as the correction of bunions. Present units are just not powerful enough to cut through bone.

I develop lots of callus on the bottom of my feet. Is there any way to prevent this painful condition?

A. Callus is caused by abnormal friction on the skin of the bottom of your foot. One way to reduce this friction is to try wearing an anti-friction insole such as a Spenco®. Regular removal of built-up callus tissue with a pumice stone may also be helpful. If you still have problems after this, see your podiatrist.

The Foot Health Test

1. Do your feet often feel cold?

   Yes ✓____ (2 points)
   Sometimes ____ (1 point)
   No ____ (0 points)

2. How high a heel do you usually wear?

   Flat ____ (1 point)
   one inch ____ (0 points)
   two inches ____ (1 point)
   three inches or more ____ (2 points)

3. Describe your arch height?

   Low arch ✓____ (2 points)
   Medium arch ____ (0 points)
   High arch ____ (1 point)

4. Which of your parents have had foot problems?

   Neither parent ____ (0 points)
   one parent ____ (1 point)
   Both parents ____ (2 points)

5. Are you a diabetic?

   Yes ____ (2 points)
   No ____ (0 points)

6. Describe your body type

   Thin ____ (0 points)
   Medium ____ (1 point)
   Heavy ____ (2 points

7. What is the skin condition of your feet?

   Dry ✓____ (1 point)

Neither dry nor moist _____ (0 points)
Moist or sweaty _____ (2 points)

8. Which is your longest toe?

The big toe _____ (0 points)
The second toe _____ (2 points)

9. Do your feet often "burn"?

Yes _____ (2 points)
Sometimes _____ (1 point)
No _____ (0 points)

10. How often do you participate in sports that involve running?

Seldom or never _____ (0 points)
Once or twice a week _____ (1 point)
At least three times a week _____ (2 points)

11. Do you have bunions?

Yes _____ (2 points)
No _____ (0 points

12. Do you have hammertoes?

Yes _____ (2 points)
No _____ (0 points)

13. Are your toenails thickened or ingrown?

Yes _____ (2 points)
No _____ (0 points)

14. Do you suffer from corns or calluses?

Yes _____ (2 points)
Sometimes _____ (1 point)
No _____ (0 points)

15. Do your feet ache at the end of the day?

Always _____ (2 points)
Sometimes _____ (1 point)
No _____ (0 points)

Answer key to foot health test

1. Cold feet are a sign of poor circulation. Since the blood vessels in the feet are among the smallest in the body, they are among the first to react to decreased circulation.

2. The best heel height for most people is about one inch. Flat heels are unsatisfactory because in most people they cause the knees to hyperextend. As heel height exceeds two inches, increased pressure is put on the ball of the foot. Above three inches, ankle instability becomes an additional problem.

3. Low arches are often a result of pronated or "flatfeet." High arched feet serve as poor shock absorbers. Medium arched feet seem to function best.

4. Heredity is a factor in many foot conditions. Bunions, hammertoes, gout, and flatfeet are among the many foot problems passed on from one generation to the next. Heredity is also a factor in metabolic diseases such as gout and diabetes which affect the foot.

5. The feet of diabetic patients are particularly prone to infection and ulceration. Diabetics require the regular care of a podiatrist.

6. The feet must bear your entire body weight. Excess weight acts to "break down" the structure of the feet. Flatfeet, heel spurs, and plantar fasciitis are common in overweight individuals.

7. Moist foot skin provides an excellent medium for the growth of bacteria and fungi. Dry skin leads to cracking and fissuring of the feet. Ideally, the skin of the feet should be neither moist nor dry.

8. The foot generally functions best if the big toe is the longest. The big toe acts as a propulsive lever in walking. Those with a short big toe (Morton's foot) tend to suffer from more foot problems.

9. Burning feet are generally a sign of excessive friction on the bottom of the feet. This is usually associated with callus formation. Burning feet can also indicate systemic problems such as pernicious anemia.

10. Running is a great way to build up cardiovascular fitness. Unfortunately, it is also very tough on the feet. With each step a runner hits the ground with three times his body weight.

11. Bunions are a sign of badly pronated feet. They are often painful and make shoe fitting difficult.

12. Hammertoes indicate poor foot structure and function. They often result in corns on the top of the toes.

13. Ingrown toenails are painful and potentially a source of a dangerous infection. Thickened toenails are unattractive and make shoe fitting difficult.

14. Corns and calluses are a result of abnormal friction during walking. This can be a result of poor foot structure or poorly fitting shoes.

15. Chronic aching feet are a sign of fatigue due to poor foot function. It is normal for your feet to ache occasionally, especially after a long walk.

Evaluating your score:

0–7 points. Your feet are in good condition.

8–12 points. Your feet are in fair condition. See a podiatrist periodically.

13 or more points. Your feet are in poor condition. See a podiatrist regularly.

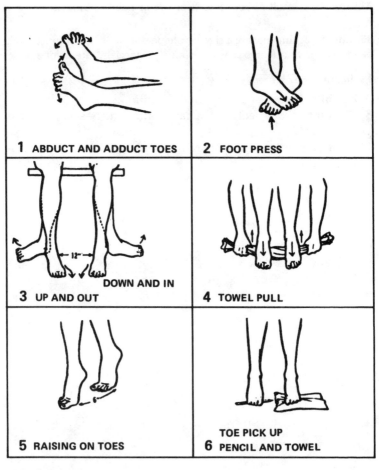

1 ABDUCT AND ADDUCT TOES

2 FOOT PRESS

DOWN AND IN
3 UP AND OUT

4 TOWEL PULL

5 RAISING ON TOES

TOE PICK UP
6 PENCIL AND TOWEL

Exercises 1 to 6:

Move ankles, feet and toes slowly through these exercises.

Exercises 7 and 8:

Raise one leg at a time, lowering slowly. Then raise both legs together and lower slowly.

164

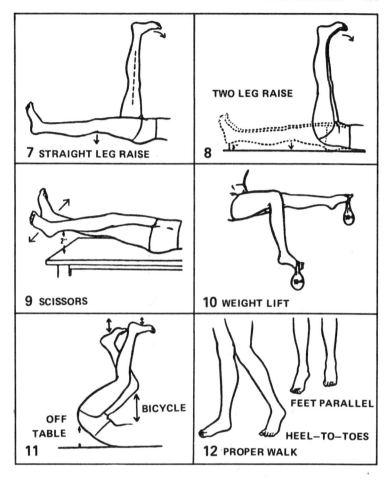

Exercise 9:

Raise legs up two inches from floor or bed and slowly cross and uncross them.

Exercise 10:

With ten pound weight across foot, elevate alternately the right leg, then the left leg, to ninety degrees.

Exercise 12:

When walking, keep feet parallel and finish step on the toes (not on ball of foot).

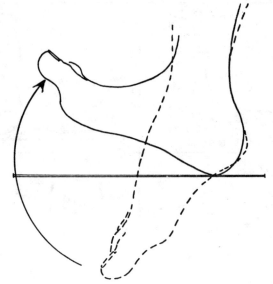

Dorsiflexion of the foot

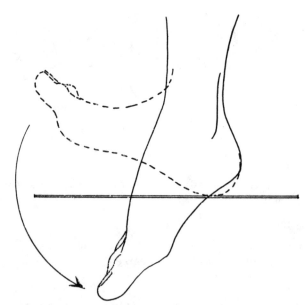

Plantarflexion of the foot

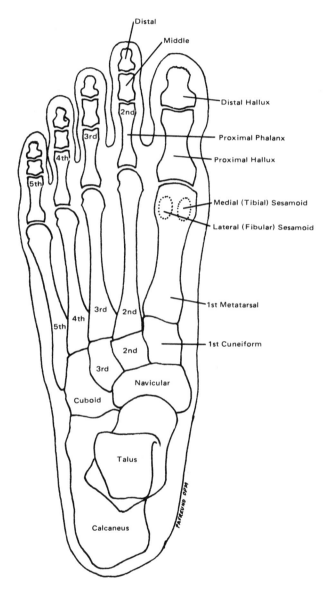

Distal

Middle

2nd

3rd

4th

5th

Distal Hallux

Proximal Phalanx

Proximal Hallux

Medial (Tibial) Sesamoid

Lateral (Fibular) Sesamoid

1st Metatarsal

1st Cuneiform

3rd

4th

5th

2nd

2nd

3rd

Navicular

Cuboid

Talus

Calcaneus

Dorsal View

Medial View

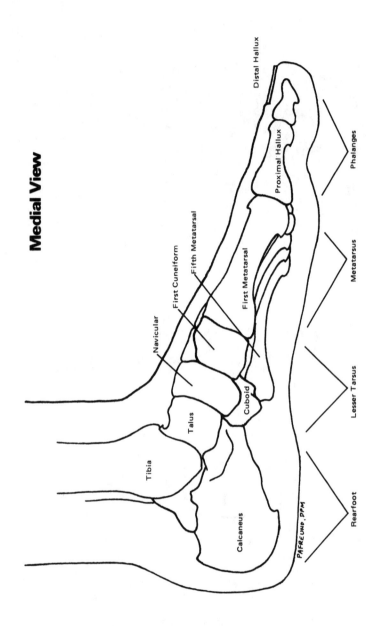

Distal Hallux

Proximal Hallux

Fifth Metatarsal

First Cuneiform

First Metatarsal

Navicular

Cuboid

Talus

Tibia

Calcaneus

PAFREUND, DPM

Phalanges

Metatarsus

Lesser Tarsus

Rearfoot

Lateral View

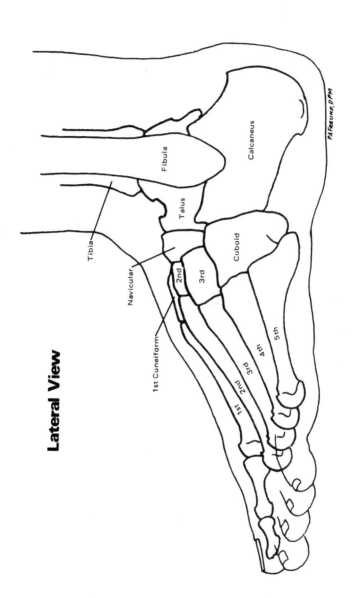

Glossary

ABNORMAL PRONATION. A flattening motion of the foot which leads to a "collapsing" of the arch. This destructive force can lead to such conditions as bunions, flatfeet, and heel spurs.

ACHILLES TENDINITIS. An inflammation of the large tendon of the calf muscle at the point where it connects to the heel bone.

ACROCYNANOSIS. A condition in which the toes and fingers assume a bluish tone due to a spasm of small arteries.

ACUTE. Rapid onset of a condition.

AMBULATORY FOOT SURGERY. Foot surgery, usually performed in a doctor's office which allows for immediate walking.

ANHIDROSIS. Excessively dry feet.

APOPHYSITIS. Irritation of the growth plate of a bone. This commonly occurs in the heel bone of active children and is known as Sever's apophysitis.

ARCH. (Longitudinal). The inside area of the foot extending from the heel to the metatarsals.

ARCH SUPPORT. A shoe insert designed to help support the arch.

ARTERIOSCLEROSIS. A condition resulting in the thickening, narrowing, and loss of elasticity of the inside of arteries. Arteriosclerosis is commonly known as "hardening of the arteries" and occurs frequently in the elderly.

ARTHRITIS. A general term applied to any disease which affects the joints.

ARTHROPLASTY. A surgical procedure involving remodeling of a joint.

ASTEOTOSIS. A decrease in the size of the fat pad of the foot.

ATHLETE'S FOOT. A condition caused by a fungal infection. Fungi are parasitic plant-like organisms which like to live in moist, dark and warm places. Athlete's foot is characterized by itchy, peeling skin. Sometimes small fluid filled sacs are present.

BALL OF THE FOOT. The area behind the toes on the bottom surface of the foot. Anatomically this area lies just below the metatarsal bones.

BROMHIDROSIS. Foul odor usually caused by the action of sweat, bacteria, yeast and fungus on the skin.

BUNION. (Also known as hallux valgus or hallux abducto valgus). This is a deformity which occurs at the big toe joint. A large bony prominence is usually present. As this deformity develops, the big toe often angles toward the outside of the foot.

BUNIONECTOMY. A surgical procedure for the correction of a bunion deformity.

BUNIONETTE. See TAILOR'S BUNION.

BURSITIS. Inflammation of a bursa, a balloon-like sac which surrounds a joint and fills with fluids in response to joint irritation.

CALLUS. A thickening of skin which occurs in response to excessive pressure. Calluses occur on large areas of the sole of the foot.

CAPSULE. The fibrous tissue surrounding a joint.

CAPSULITIS. Irritation of a capsule.

CAPSULOTOMY. A surgical procedure in which a joint capsule is cut. Capsulotomies are usually performed in conjunction with tenotomies.

CALCANEUS. The heel bone.

CAVUS FOOT. A foot with a high arch.

CELLULITIS. A spreading inflammation of tissue, usually due to infection.

CHIROPODIST. The predecessors of modern podiatrists. This term is still used in the United Kingdom and elsewhere.

CHONDROMALACIA. A knee condition resulting from uneven wearing of the cartilage under the knee cap. This condition is also referred to as "runner's knee" and can result from improper foot function.

CLUB NAIL. A thickened and deformed nail. Club nails may be the result of a chronic fungus infection or trauma to the nail.

CLUBFOOT. A congenital deformity of the foot requiring immediate treatment.

CONGENITAL. Present at birth.

COOKIES. Children's arch supports which were popular in the 1940s and 1950s.

CORN. A thickening of the skin which occurs in response to excessive pressure. Corns generally occur on the toes. Soft corns occur between the toes.

COUNTER. The back part of the shoe which surrounds the heel.

CUTICLE. The skin covering the back part of a nail.

DERMATITIS. Irritation of the skin.

DIABETES MELLITUS. A metabolic disease in which the body cannot properly transfer blood sugar into body tissues. Diabetics suffer from vascular problems and require routine foot care.

DORSI-FLEXION. An upward motion of a body part. (Think of what happens to your foot when you bring your "toes toward your nose.")

DORSUM. The top of the foot.

ERYTHRASMA. An infection caused by a plant-like organism called cornyebacterium minutissimum. Erythrasma usually occurs between the toes and is often confused with athlete's foot.

ERYTHROMELALGIA. A rare condition characterized by increased temperature, redness, and a burning sensation in both feet.

EQUINUS. A condition in which there is a limitation in the ability of the foot to dorsiflex. This is often associated with tight calf muscles.

EXOSTOSIS. An extra accumulation of bone such as a calcium deposit. An exostosis is sometimes referred to as a spur.

FISSURE. A crack in the skin. These are most often found between the toes and around the heel area.

GOUT. A metabolic disease in which excess uric acid accumulates in the body and precipitates in the big toe joint causing sudden pain.

HALLUX LIMITUS. This is the early stage of an arthritic condition affecting the big toe joint. A small accumulation of bone around the joint limits the normal motion of the joint.

HALLUX RIGIDUS. This is the late stage of an arthritic condition affecting the big toe joint. A large accumulation of extra bone surrounding the joint restricts normal joint motion.

HALLUX VALGUS. See BUNION.

HAMMERTOE. A deformity in which the toe "buckles up" with the "knuckle" in a raised position. This subjects the top of the toe to corn formation.

HANGNAIL. A piece of tissue "hanging" loose from the side of a nail.

HEEL LIFT. A piece of material added below the heel. This can either be placed in the shoe or built on to the heel of the shoe.

HEEL SPUR. A condition in which a piece of bone is gradually "pulled" from the heel bone by taut plantar ligaments which attach to it. Abnormal collapsing of the arch of the foot is the major cause of this painful condition.

HEMATOMA. An accumulation of blood found below the skin or nail (subungual hematoma).

HYPERHIDROSIS. A condition in which the skin sweats excessively.

HYPERKERATOSIS. An excessive build-up of skin such as occurs in corns and calluses.

INGROWN TOENAIL. A painful condition in which the outside edge of a nail presses into the adjoining flesh which surrounds it.

INSOLE. A shoe insert usually added to provide better shock absorption.

INTERMITTENT CLAUDICATION. Sharp pain which occurs in the calf muscles during walking. This pain occurs at measurable intervals (such as every two blocks) and is relieved by rest. Intermittent claudication is a sign of poor circulation.

INTRACTABLE PLANTAR KERATOMA (IPK). A painful callus-like lesion found on the bottom of the foot, usually underneath a metatarsal bone (at the ball of the foot). An IPK forms because one or more metatarsal bones is structurally lower than the others.

ITIS. A suffix meaning irritated or inflamed.

LASER SURGERY. The use of a powerful beam of concentrated light as a means of cutting or destroying tissue.

LAST. A model of the foot from which shoes are made.

LESION. Any change in the normal appearance of tissue. Extra build-ups of skin such as corns or calluses are considered lesions. So are cuts, abrasions or ulcerations of skin.

LIGAMENT. Strong fibers of tissue that connect one bone to another.

MACERATION. A condition in which the skin becomes soggy due to a prolonged exposure to moisture.

MATRIX. The area at the back of a nail (below the cuticle) from which the nail grows.

METATARSALS. The five long bones of the foot. They begin in the middle of the foot and end near the back part of the toes.

MICROSURGERY. Surgery performed with the aid of a microscope. Microsurgery is used to reattach severed body parts.

MINIMAL INCISION SURGERY. Surgery performed through a small skin incision.

MORTON'S FOOT. A structural condition in which the big toe is shorter than the second toe. This may predispose one to foot problems.

MORTON'S NEUROMA. A benign nerve tumor usually found between the third and fourth metatarsal bones. This condition causes pain which radiates to the third and fourth toes and is aggravated by the wearing of narrow shoes.

MYCOTIC. Fungus infected.

NAIL SULCUS. The skin groove surrounding a nail.

NEUROMA. See MORTON'S NEUROMA.

ONYCHOMYCOTIC. A fungus infected nail.

ORTHOTIC. A custom-made shoe insert designed to help you walk better in the same manner that eyeglasses allow you to see better. Orthotics are commonly made of leather, plastic, or metal. Orthotics are useful in the treatment of many foot conditions including flatfeet, abnormal pronation, Achilles tendinitis, plantar fasciitis, and knee pain.

OS CALCUS. An old name for the heel bone.

OSTEOARTHRITIS. A type of arthritis resulting from the excessive wear and tear of joint surfaces.

OSTEOTOMY. The surgical cutting of a bone.

PES PLANUS. A low arched foot.

PLANTAR. The bottom surface of the foot, known as the sole.

PLANTAR-FLEXION. A downward motion.

PLANTAR FASCIITIS. Irritation of the ligaments of the arch of the foot. This condition often leads to heel spurs.

PLANTAR WART. (Also known as verruca or papilloma). A benign skin growth occurring on the bottom (plantar) of the foot. Warts are caused by a virus infection. They are most commonly contracted by walking barefoot on a wet abrasive surface such as a shower stall of a health club.

PODIATRIST. A physician of the foot. Licensed as a Doctor of Podiatric Medicine to diagnose and treat (medically, orthopedically, surgically) any disorder affecting the foot.

POROMETRIC. A man-made material that "breathes."

PRONATION. The normal motion the foot undergoes in adjusting to the ground. The foot is extremely flexible during pronation. See also ABNORMAL PRONATION.

PROUD FLESH. See PYOGENIC GRANULOMA.

PYOGENIC GRANULOMA. Chronically infected tissue, commonly associated with ingrown toenails.

RAYNAUD'S DISEASE. A condition in which the fingers and toes turn white, blue and red in response to cold weather or emotional stress.

REFLEXOLOGY. A branch of holistic medicine. Proponents claim that specific points on the foot correspond to different body parts. They contend that applying pressure to these areas can bring relief to diseased organs. There is little scientific data to support these claims.

SESAMOID. A bone found within a tendon. Two small sesamoids are normally found in the tendon beneath the first metatarsal bone.

SEVER'S APOPHYSITIS. See APOPHYSITIS.

SHANK. A hard piece of material (usually steel) added to the arch area of a shoe to provide additional support.

SHIN SPLINTS. A painful condition resulting in irritation of the musculature of the lower leg.

SOFT CORN. A thickening of the skin between two toes.

SPICULE. A small, often sharp nail fragment which can pierce the nail sulcus causing an ingrown nail.

SPRAIN. An injury of a joint, usually involving local ligaments and tendons.

STRAIN. An injury to a muscle, usually due to overuse.

SULCUS. See NAIL SULCUS.

SUPINATION. A motion which causes the foot to act as a rigid lever. Supination is the opposite of pronation.

TAILOR'S BUNION. An enlargement of the metatarsal bone at the outside part of the foot (the fifth metatarsal).

TENDON. A band of tissue connecting a muscle to another structure (usually a bone).

TENDINITIS. An inflamed tendon.

TENOTOMY. The surgical cutting of a tendon.

TINEA PEDIS. A fungus infection of the foot.

TRICEPS SURAE. The calf muscles.

ULCER. An open sore.

ULTRASOUND. A form of physical therapy using vibrating sound waves.

VAMP. The front part of a shoe covering the top of the foot.

VERRUCAE. See plantar wart.

WART. See plantar wart.

XERODERMA. Excessive dryness of the skin.

ZONE THERAPY. See *reflexology*.

Component Societies
of the American Podiatry
Association

ALABAMA PODIATRY ASSOCIATION. Donald S. Provenzano, 525 S. 3rd St., Gadsden AL 35901.

ARIZONA PODIATRY ASSOCIATION. James E. Stocker, 3555 W. Greenway Rd., Phoenix, AZ 85023.

ARKANSAS PODIATRY ASSOCIATION. John A. Werner, 2912 Rogers Ave., Ste. B, Fort Smith, AR 72901.

CALIFORNIA PODIATRIC MEDICAL ASSOCIATION. Robert O. Johns (Executive Director), 26 O'Farrell St, Ste. 200, San Francisco, CA 94108.

COLORADO PODIATRY ASSOCIATION. Mr. Leo Boyle (Executive Director), 1726 Champa, Ste. 216, Denver, CO 80202.

CONNECTICUT PODIATRY ASSOCIATION. Mr. Angelo J. DeMio (Executive Director), 48 Crest St., Wethersfield, CT 06109.

DELAWARE, PODIATRY SOCIETY OF. David S. Guggenheim, 2018 Naamas Rd., Ste. Al, Wilmington, DE 19810.

DISTRICT OF COLUMBIA, PODIATRY SOCIETY OF THE. Mr. Larry I. Shane, (Executive Director), 1729 Glastonberry Rd., Potomac, MD 20854.

FEDERAL SERVICE, ASSOCIATION OF PODIATRISTS IN. LTC Dan W. Hunt, (Executive Director), OSC Box 250, WRAMC, Washington, DC 20012.

FLORIDA PODIATRY ASSOCIATION. William D. Ownes, (Executive Director), 325 John Knox Rd., L-250, Tallahassee, FL 32303.

GEORGIA PODIATRIC MEDICAL ASSOCIATION, INC. Wesley L. Daniel, 416 Broad St., SE, Gainsville, GA 30501.

HAWAII PODIATRY ASSOCIATION. Theodore G. York, 615 Piikoi St., 11401, Honolulu, HI 96814.

IDAHO PODIATRY ASSOCIATION. Charles F. Call, 1587 E. 17th St., Idaho Falls, ID 83401.

ILLINOIS PODIATRY SOCIETY. Mr. Norm Netko (Executive Director), 65 E. South Water St., Ste. 1110, Chicago, IL 60601.

INDIANA STATE PODIATRY ASSOCIATION. Mr. Ronald W. Wuensch (Executive Consultant), 514 Illinois Bldg., Des Moines, IA 50309.

KANSAS PODIATRY ASSOCIATION. Mr. Wayne Probasco (Executive Director), 615 S. Topeka, Topeka, KS 6603.

KENTUCKY PODIATRY ASSOCIATION. Mr. E. C. Stivers, Jr. (Executive Director), 1705 Bardstown Rd., Louisville, KY 40205.

LOUISIANA STATE PODIATRY ASSOCIATION. Steven J. Watson, 108 Smart Pl., Slidell, LA 70458.

MAINE PODIATRY ASSOCIATION. Roy B. Corbin, 276 State St., Bangor, ME 04401.

MARYLAND PODIATRY ASSOCIATION. Mr. Larry I. Shane (Executive Director), 1729 Glastonberry Rd., Potomac, MD 20854.

MASSACHUSETTS PODIATRY SOCIETY, INC. Thomas F. Connolly (Executive Director), 14 Beacon St., Rm. 404, Boston, MA 02108.

MICHIGAN STATE PODIATRY ASSOCIATION. LTC David P. Williams (Executive Vice-President), 412 W. Ottawa St., Lansing, MI 48933.

MINNESOTA PODIATRY ASSOCIATION. H. Michael Lee, 29 9th Ave. N, Hopkins, MN 55343.

MISSISSIPPI PODIATRY ASSOCIATION. John W. Benus, 4311 Chico Rd., Pascagoula, MS 39567.

MISSOURI PODIATRY ASSOCIATION. Mr. William A. Spencer (Executive Director), 215 E. Capitol, PO Box 1733, Jefferson City, MO 65102.

MONTANA PODIATRY ASSOCIATION. Robert D. Phillips, 2526 12th Ave S, Great Falls, MT 59405.

NEBRASKA PODIATRY ASSOCIATION. Ms. Jean Muntz (Executive Secretary), 1910 S. 44th St., Omaha, NE 68105.

NEVADA PODIATRY SOCIETY. Carl B. Smith, 3376 S. Eastern Ave., Ste. 166, Las Vegas, NV 89109.

NEW HAMPSHIRE PODIATRY ASSOCIATION. Stanley A. Gorgol, 198 Main St., Salem, NH 03079.

NEW JERSEY PODIATRY SOCIETY. Mr. Irving J. Tecker (Executive Director), Blason II, 505 S. Lenola Rd., Moorestown, NJ 08057.

NEW MEXICO PODIATRY SOCIETY. Ms. Doris Conley (Executive Director), 1400 Catron SE, Albuquerque, NM 87123.

NEW YORK, THE PODIATRY SOCIETY OF THE STATE OF. Stan Matek (Executive Director), 875 Avenue of the Americas, New York, NY 10001.

NORTH CAROLINA PODIATRY SOCIETY. C. Jeff Mauney, 89 N. Lafayette St., PO Box 1801, Shelby, NC 28150.

NORTH DAKOTA ASSOCIATION OF PODIATRISTS. Omer H. Welna, 1402 25th St., S. Fargo, ND 58103.

OHIO PODIATRY ASSOCIATION. Mrs. Jeannine Gaston (Executive Director), 2041 Riverside Dr., Columbus, OH 43221.

OKLAHOMA PODIATRY ASSOCIATION. Mr. Jack J. Francis (Executive Director), PO Box 55441, Tulsa, OK 74155.

178   **Foot Talk**

OREGON PODIATRY ASSOCIATION. David M. Wellikoff, 1715 S. Baker St., McMinnville, OR 97128.

PENNSYLVANIA PODIATRY ASSOCIATION. Mr. Matthew M. Shook, Jr. (Executive Director), 757 Poplar Church Rd., Camp Hill, PA 17011.

PUERTO RICO PODIATRY ASSOCIATION. Jose Romeu Garcia, Cond. San Martin, Pa 23-Ste. 511, Santurce, PR 00909.

RHODE ISLAND PODIATRY SOCIETY. Peter J. Lewis, 1087 Warwick Ave., Warwick, RI 02888.

SOUTH CAROLINA PODIATRY ASSOCIATION. William McAninch, 1211 Northampton Rd., Anderson, SC 29621.

SOUTH DAKOTA ASSOCIATION OF PODIATRISTS. Neil E. Skea, 505 Kansas City St., Rapid City, SD 57701.

TENNESSEE PODIATRY ASSOCIATION. William F. Lambert, 525 Two Mile Hwy., Ste. 3, Goodlettsville, TN 37072.

TEXAS PODIATRY ASSOCIATION. Maryvenice E. Stewart (Executive Director), 5017 Bull Creek Rd., Austin, TX 78731.

UTAH PODIATRY ASSOCIATION. Steven D. Smith, 144 South 7th East, Salt Lake City, Utah 84121.

VERMONT PODIATRY ASSOCIATION. Raymond Mariani (Executive Director), 42 Western Ave., Brattleboro, VT 05301.

VIRGINIA, INC. PODIATRY SOCIETY OF. Ms. Jennifer Ayers (Corresponding Secretary), PO Box 1417, Ste. A-42, Alexandria, VA 22313.

WASHINGTON STATE PODIATRY ASSOCIATION. Ben Scapa, 15630 Redmond Way, Redmond, WA 98052.

WEST VIRGINIA PODIATRY SOCIETY. Roy C. Harmon, 55 15th St., Wheeling, WV 26003.

WISCONSIN SOCIETY OF PODIATRIC MEDICINE. Kevin Kortsch (Executive Director), 2500 N. Mayfair Rd., Wauwatosa, WI 53226.

WYOMING PODIATRY SOCIETY. John W. Aaron, III, 423 5th St., Rock Springs, WY 82901.

Index

179